Contents

Introduction

My Seizure Poem

PART 1 – About Epilepsy

Chapter 1 – About Epilepsy
Chapter 2 – My Other Conditions

PART 2 – My Story

Chapter 1   – In the Beginning
Chapter 2   – An Angry Teenager
Chapter 3   – The Halls
Chapter 4   – Moving On
Chapter 5   – Glasgow
Chapter 6   – Back Home
Chapter 7   – The Test Results
Chapter 8   – London
Chapter 9   – A New Adventure
Chapter 10 – Making New Friends
Chapter 11 – The Consent Form
Chapter 12 – Surgery
Chapter 13 – Recovery
Chapter 14 – Research and Progress
Chapter 15 – Family Reunions
Chapter 16 – Living with Epilepsy and the Perceptions of Others

PART 3 – Breaking the Stigma

Chapter 17   – Campaigns and Charities
Chapter 18   – Self Employment

Conclusion
Glossary
Disclaimer
Useful Links and Organisations

Introduction

In historic times people with epilepsy were seen as either gods or demons, or simply an embarrassment to their family. As a result people with any kind of neurological condition or illness were simply locked away in what were known as asylums or mental institutions.

Today we know them as respite care or care homes; or places where people with a variety of medical conditions go to get help and support.

But has anything really changed?

Ignorance still continues in a world of ignorance, and discrimination in a society where epilepsy is simply misunderstood and stigmatised. Discrimination is a constant problem for those with this condition.

However, scientists and doctors now work together with patients who willingly give up their time to assist with research in the hope that future generations can learn from and understand their experiences, and progress towards a change if not a cure.

This is why I have written about it and why everything I have mentioned has a place in my story. If it was not for the experiences I have encountered and the people I have met along the way I would not have been able to make this book possible so thank you.

I have no regrets and do not hold any resentment for the past nor any of the experiences I have had so far. Every obstacle and journey I have encountered was relevant, even though at times I rebelled and felt I was wasting my time or was walking around in circles.

My name is Jolene Modd, I was born full term in Davyhulme hospital on the fourteenth of august 1978. I am told I was born small for my size. I was 4lbs and 2ounces. I was born stressed. The hospital believed me to be premature because of my low birth weight.

I was an intelligent child who never complained and did not experience my first convulsion until the age of two years old. I learned to have patience though I was often frustrated that what I wanted simply did not happen fast enough. Eventually I learned the lesson that I was simply ahead of my time and at times I was simply not ready for the types of careers I wanted.

My spirituality helped me to learn that eventually when the time was right I would get what I wanted regardless of disability. I believed that it was up to me to change my life. I was still in control regardless of my condition.

My Seizure poem

Sometimes I'm Chatting to friends or family,
Walking the streets, going about my business quite happily,
Then I wake up, I don't know what's happened,
My mind is all messed up; my head went all fuzzy,
The room went all white, the sun I was aware just how yellow and bright.
For a while a short second I was transported somewhere else,
I was transported to another land, another time,
Though it felt my spirit had been jolted from itself.
Even though I panicked, even though I was scared,
Something inside me just did not care.

People around me asking are you ok?
Seem to be concerned about me; however they seem to be ok,
Though they are strangers to me, they are freaking me out.
I just want to sleep, I will sleep just right where I am.
Though I feel confused right now,
I just do not care, not sure where I am,
Though I know I'm scared, though I am not sure why.

I just don't care, my instinct is telling me to get away,
To run away from here, but where,
Where to, where do I go?
I'm not sure of my surroundings right now,
Confused and disorientated, I don't know where I am,
Just what was I doing before, where was I going,
As I get up to walk away in the wrong direction,
I hear someone say, come back, the ambulance is on its way.

Apparently I hurt my head; I need to get it checked.
Though I have no memory, no pain, and no sensation,
I am fine now remembering where I am.

No need for any ambulance I can send them on their way,
Tomorrow I will have a headache perhaps a vivid memory of today,
For now of course I need some clarity as I come round,
Someone to sit with me, just tell me I am sound.
It was only a seizure, not much else, only a seizure
A seizure it may be, though frightened and scared,
A big deal it was to me.

PART 1

ABOUT EPILEPSY

This section of the book provides background information about epilepsy and other conditions that I suffer from, and may help you to understand my story more fully.

However, if you would rather read PART 2 – MY STORY first then please do.

Chapter 1

About Epilepsy

Over the years I have found there have been many assumptions made about myself, especially during a seizure, and with regard to my epilepsy, my anxiety and fainting attacks.

I found that as I embarked on my basic first aid training I was only ever given the basics when it came to epilepsy awareness training. In employment environments I was usually left to inform staff and manage myself which usually consisted of meetings with human resources or my supervisor. I found it was only when I had a seizure that actual training came in to effect.

So before I tell you my story, I am going to provide some details about the different types of seizures and what to do when a seizure, fit, black out or fainting attack occurs. I found epilepsy training to be beneficial although regardless of how many times I did the course I was constantly doing refreshers and reading up on material because of the amount of research and new material that was constantly been updated and becoming available. **(See the BMA for further details)**

So what happens to the brain during a seizure? Well a seizure is like an electrical storm going off in the head. What happens to the affected person outside on or around the body all depends on which part of the brain encounters this wave of electricity or storm. The brain is a sensitive organ and can easily be damaged though not easily repaired. A seizure can last anything from a few seconds to 15 minutes, although the recovery time can take all day depending on the type of seizure and how badly the person has been affected. After effects can be anything from an anxiety attack to a headache. Some people have seizures that only affect one small part of the brain and medication controls their seizures well. Others have many different types of seizures which can often lead to other conditions such as anxiety, O.C.D, depression, autism, and on occasion learning disabilities which could be a result of long term medication (side effects) or the amount of seizures a person has encountered over the years and the damage this caused to the brain or the length of time spent in a seizure.

What to do if you experience someone having a seizure

- **Protect the person from injury – remove any harmful objects from nearby. Cushion their head with a pillow, blanket, coat or the person's handbag.**
- **Look for an epilepsy identity card or identity jewellery or any other form of identification that might help to tell you more about the person's condition.**
- **Aid their breathing by gently placing them in the recovery position once the seizure has finished and always stay with the person until recovery is complete.**

- **Be calm and reassuring** I know from personal experience with my seizures that depending on the person's reaction I can be verbally aggressive, very assertive or will respond accordingly. I have been chucked out of shops and come round to find myself with a security guard and this can be rather frightening. I have wanted to just get out of the place or situation I was in. I've found myself with or in an ambulance, and even the police in some strange situations.

- **Never restrain the person's movements,** hold them down or put anything in the person's mouth, unless you want to get your fingers bitten off.

- **Never try to move them unless they are or you are in danger.**

- For example if you are both on the road, or the railway it is important to get the person to a safe place. Common sense is important here. sometime asking the cars to stop or closing down the road or diverting traffic would be a more appropriate option. **Your safety comes first.**

- One rule I have never quite understood is **never give them anything to eat or drink until they are fully recovered** though I can understand this rule for status epilepsy. It takes me a while to recover. I never want anything to eat or drink after a seizure. I'm always hungry or thirsty building up to a seizure.

- **Do not Attempt to bring them round yourself don't make any sense to me.** I always recover faster if i can feel someone playing with my ears or can hear direct communication. As long as you are trained and have put the person in the recovery position and they are not in any danger as far as i am concerned you have saved a person's life. Always ring for the emergency service not that the person will want or need to go to hospital but as a long as you stay with that person and are reassuring then you have saved the person's life. I suppose the message here is if in doubt call them out. which brings me on to the next so called rule.

- Only call for an ambulance if you know it is the person's **first seizure**, or the seizure continues for **more than five minutes**, if **one tonic-clonic seizure follows another without the person regaining consciousness between seizures**, or if the person is **injured** during the seizure, or if you have reason to believe the person needs urgent medical attention. **For a complex partial,**(seizures affecting a larger part of the brain) **simple partial** (seizures confined to a small part of the brain) or **absence seizure**

- (Also known as Petit Mal attacks, short blank spells), the person is not always in any danger and does not always require an ambulance. though i imagine without epilepsy first aid which is separate from basic first aid or some experience in epilepsy I guess it would be hard to tell.

Epilepsy is now broken down into five groups:-

(1) **Generalised** seizures,

(2) **Partial** seizures,

(3) **Idiopathic, Simple Partial** epilepsy

(4) **Symptomatic** epilepsy which is a new type and usually develops when there is a structural abnormality in the brain

(5) **Cryptogenic** epilepsy which is also a new category.

Generalised seizures can be anything from **absence seizures, atonic seizures, tonic seizures, myoclonic seizures** and even **tonic clonic seizures**. First aid also varies depending on what type of seizure the person is experiencing. A person experiencing a seizure does not always require an ambulance, sometimes they simply require you to stay with them till they come round and offer them some reassurance. However there are certain times during a seizure when an ambulance is necessary (see above). generalised seizures can begin in both half's of the brain at once without warning.

In **partial** epilepsy people will experience **simple partial** or **complex partial** seizures in which again the symptoms can vary.

Living with Epilepsy

Some people have difficulty coming to terms with their diagnoses. Others have difficulty getting proper diagnoses in the early stages or first few years of epilepsy. Then there are people out there who have difficulty just living with epilepsy. This could be anything from the **stigmas** to the **attitudes** or the day to day **challenges** in life.

I know because I have faced them all.

Over time epilepsy gets worse. This could be due to age or memory deterioration. With age everyone can look forward to a decline in memory or can say they know someone who suffers from Alzheimer's or dementia. However a person with epilepsy will find that as the signals in the brain weaken or the brain shrinks, or the seizures find other parts of the brain to attack, their memory declines. This can manifest its self in many ways, for example; problems with long or short memory, poor visual memory recall or problems with remembering faces and names and problems with speech; or dementia, Alzheimer's, depression or other mental health issues. Over time these issues or health problems all become part of epilepsy's decline.

Mental illness, mental health and other neurological conditions can become a vicious circle. There are many specialists out there and consultants that work together to help patients and sufferers along with various charities. However not many people understand or are aware of the full implications of what it is like living with epilepsy.

I have found a range of support groups and organisations that have been growing over the years to help raise awareness and support people although there is still a huge majority that are not aware of what it is like from the perspective of the person living with the condition or from the family or friends' point of view. Anyone who has watched a person suffer with epilepsy goes through the same experience, and lives with epilepsy also. It is not just the person who has epilepsy who suffers emotionally, physically and mentally, it is also the carers, friends or family members and all those who are involved in their care. It is a life sentence for anyone who gets involved which is probably why most people choose to walk away or ignore epilepsy completely.

I have found that my life sentence has been too much for me at times. There have been many times when I to have wanted to give up and end it all. What has stopped me are those people who have bothered to walk alongside me and take their time to help and support me even when I know it has been frustrating for them. I know life can be tough but I also know there are people out there who are worse off who still carry on. This knowledge and awareness is what keeps me going. There are always two sides to every story.

Chapter Two

My Other Conditions

Memory and Epilepsy

Throughout my life I have always experienced problems with my memory, concentration and focus. My mum used to send me to the shop with a small shopping list that consists of three items and I would always forget item number three. I had difficulty remembering and learning my times tables. Which I still struggle with today. At school I found learning and various classes such as English, maths and science a struggle. I still study and enjoy learning though I find these classes a challenge.

People often put this down to me being slightly dyslexic but my memory has a lot to do with it too. I have difficulty remembering when to place the letter "H" for "has" or removing the letter "h" for "as". I know when to use it in communication but due to my memory I often get confused or just can't remember. Some people say it is the amount of seizures that cause my memory problems although since carrying out my research I have found that memory problems can also be linked to depression and stress. However, I am not the only person that experiences memory problems. I found while doing research into my family history that a lot of my family also suffer from stress and memory problems and there is also history of mental health thus making anxiety and stress very common. I found that looking into my family history was helpful. Dyslexia runs in my mother's side of the family.

During a seizure my memory can be affected. I have experienced temporary amnesia, confusion and sometimes even lost part of or all of my day. I found that if I do not drink enough fluids or dehydrate then this can also cause confusion and affect my concentration and short term or long term memory. This happens because a loss of consciousness can interfere with normal brain processes, disrupting the encoding and storage of information. The confusion that can occur following a seizure can also prevent the memory from working properly. Some people with epilepsy can experience unusual electrical activity within the brain between seizures and this can also affect attention and memory functions.

People who do not understand memory and epilepsy, dementia, dyslexia or how the memory works would often make **incorrect assumptions** about me or accuse me of lying or been confused.

Memory problems can cause a range of difficulties, making it difficult to cope with everyday living, relationships and tasks. Meeting targets and just day to day activity can be quite distressing especially when people don't understand. These difficulties can cause a great deal of distress for the person affected. As well as friends and family members. For me I had difficulty concentrating in work, remembering names and faces or phone numbers. Mornings can be quite difficult for me although I might wake up early I do not have the energy to get up, get dressed and get out before eight **AM,** like everyone else. Rushing in the morning is most likely to cause stress to the brain and trigger brain fog or bring on a seizure. Unlike everyone else my brain needs time to come round regardless of how awake my body is. Sometimes whilst recovering from a seizure I would often forget where I was or have no memory of my location or what I was doing beforehand. Sometimes it would take me five or ten minutes before I could even speak or communicate with the person who happened to be present or with me at the time of my recovery. If a person tries to force me to do anything or asks me any questions during this time; because I am still aware of my surroundings though not quite sure of what is going on. I can become frustrated due to my inability to verbally communicate. It is not just visual memory and spacial memory, my verbal memory is also affected during this time. However, while a memory problem cannot be cured due to the cells being eaten away through deterioration, it *is* possible to adapt to having memory impairment and live a relatively normal life.

Neutropenia

As well as having memory difficulties i also have a diagnosis of neutropenia. Neutropenia is a condition that happens when the level of neutrophils in the blood drop below 1000/cmm (per cubic millimetre).
Neutrophils are blood cells that are produced in the marrow, or core of the bones. Blood normally contains 2500 to 9900 neutrophils/cmm. My white blood count was also low 2.7 (3.7 – 11.0) i would often have test done to check my blood count.

Neutrophils are very important because they fight infection. It is important for a person with a weak immune system or neurological condition to drink plenty of fluids because dehydration can lead to the brain breaking down and not functioning properly. I have found that during my menstrual cycle if I did not drink plenty of fluids then I was likely to have an increase in seizures especially on a warm day. I often have a dry mouth with my medication but if I do not drink plenty of fluids then I feel faint anyway.

There are three main types of neutropenia and over the years I have been diagnosed with them all. When I was eight years old I was diagnosed with **idiopathic neutropenia** due to the fact that I had a white cell deficiency after coming out with blotches or red sores on my body. I had a bone marrow and blood test to identify the cause and a diagnoses of neutropenia was made. The three main groups are:-

- **Congenital** which is a diagnoses from birth, where the bone marrow produces almost no Neutrophils
- **Idiopathic** which occurs at some time in life but why is not known (autoimmune neutropenia is also in this group)
- **Cyclic** which occurs from birth or occurring very early in life.

The bone marrow starts and stops producing neutrophils in a 21 day cycle and infections, mouth ulcers, and or skin infections occur when a person is at the low point in their cycle. Infections are a serious problem for all patients with neutropenia.

Having lived with neutropenia from an early age I kind of understand why so many people were over protective of me. Yes it was important to protect me against infection and injury due to the high risk of infection because of the low white blood count and weak immune system. As a child it was very difficult to understand the importance of looking after myself and taking so much care. These days i have a range of markings that pop up on my legs and arms that tell me that my blood is not circulating properly. My gums often bleed. I got used to having arguments with the dentist about whether or not I was brushing my teeth properly. With regards to the nose bleeds. It was not until 2016 that the hospital started to inform me that it was a possible allergy or migraine that could be the cause of the nose bleeds.

As an adult who now has atonic or drop down seizures with weakness to my left side, complex partial seizures with the occasional absence seizure and myoclonic jerks I often get frustrated at the length of time my body takes to heal itself and recover. I often get annoyed at myself for being so tired and in pain. I accept the injuries on the left side of my body because I understand the weakness to my left side. However when I get injuries that cannot be explained by the doctor or healed by myself simply because of tissue damage as a result of my neutropenia; I often feel the anger and frustration my mother once felt when she was taking me to the hospital herself.

I rarely hear about blood conditions on the TV unless it is a rare condition that requires a transfusion. Though I imagine there are many out there. Also it is not often I hear about how important blood is to people and what blood actually does. When we do hear about blood the image that comes to mind is leukaemia, HIV and aids. Everyone knows that blood transfusions save lives but does everyone know how blood transfusions save lives? I lack in white blood cells which fight infection and my blood does not clot so when it came to having teeth out as a child I would often go to the dental hospital and have my teeth taken out under general anaesthetic due to the fact that I would bleed a lot. When it came to having regular injections and my blood tested it was often difficult to stop the blood flow and I know of a few nurses that would often freak out and panic over the fact that they could not stop the bleeding. As I got older the blood clotting did improve although I still find today that a small cut can become easily infected or I will be dabbing it with cotton buds and antiseptic wipes for ages to stop the bleeding. When I had surgery – which I will tell you about later in this book - I had to have a blood transfusion to replace two and a half pints of blood that I lost. After the operation my blood count was normal however I still experienced problems with my gums, blood circulation, tiredness and fatigue.

Damage Limitation

Due to the body's own inability to heal its self, I have had to learn patience over the years and find ways to prevent injury or protect myself from damage because I know there is nothing much I can do about it.

Since moving into a ground floor flat I have been supplied with shower stools and chairs that are good when I feel faint or dizzy, although I often find I simply avoid doing activities that would endanger me or cause me harm if a seizure was to occur. I find that the use of chairs can often increase the risk of danger if I was to have a seizure and perhaps if I was to use the cooker or have a shower I would probably fall and injure myself anyway. It would make no difference if I was to use the props provided.

I find I do my own risk assessments and have learned to be more self-aware I do not know if that has added to my anxiety but I often found that not everyone I spoke to was interested in listening about my condition and most would often treat me differently or I would often feel belittled or manipulated in some way; so in the end I would often try to avoid conversations and go it alone.

I hope that by sharing my own experience and knowledge I can go some way to helping others by telling My Story.

PART 2 – MY STORY

Chapter One

A New Beginning

I was born on 14th August 1978 at five minutes to midnight at Park Hospital in Davyhulme, Sale, Manchester. Weighing in at just 4lbs 2oz I was born at term with a low birth weight and had a 50/50 chance of survival as I was born stressed.

Little did I know at the time what a big impact stress was going to have on my life in the future?

I was placed in an incubator for twenty one days until I was strong enough to leave hospital. I was christened whilst in hospital because of my low birth weight and small chance of survival. However I have always been a fighter and have proved this as the years have progressed. My mother recalls that I was a tiny baby who never complained and only ever woke to feed.

My mum puts my low birth weight down to the amount of stress and anxiety she herself was under and her own life style at the time. My mother was only 16 years old when my mother gave birth to me and did not even look pregnant, she was just nine stone at the time of my birth. My father on the other hand did not stick around to see me grow up. I was always told about him while I grew up in Salford, and although my father and the rest of his side of the family were living locally I did not meet him until I was fifteen years old.

I was an intelligent baby and learned to talk at an early age. I was sent to a private nursery until I was old enough to go to a public nursery. I was very self-aware and knew all my colours, animals and parts of the body from an early age. Though when it came to going outside I was quite an anxious child and would often panic and grab hold of my mother's leg afraid to let go. I had a fear or phobia of outside and loud noises though it was never diagnosed until in my early 30's that I was born partially sighted in one eye. I would often walk in front of people as though I did not see them and if anyone rolled a ball to me I would often express fear. It was not until later on in life that I learned why. A child psychologist and other doctors or consultants diagnosed me as an emotional or anxious child and I was often labelled as a worrier. It was not until later on in high school that I was given glasses for a lazy or gliding eye. Memory problems were also another concern although it was never a big issue until I left school. I noticed I often had difficulty remembering facts and lists and had problems with English and maths. I was never quite sure if this was related to my seizures or my medication. I was never diagnosed as dyslexic until I was investigated for brain surgery and memory tests were carried out.

When I reached three months old I lost a thick cheesy discharge which turned a slight pink colour. Obvious signs of blood. By the time I was nine months old my mother was concerned although my grandmother suggested that the doctor would just laugh so nothing further was ever done about it. I was an intelligent baby though frequently tired, fragile and perhaps nervous. I was very self-aware, observant and intuitive. I've always been very intuitive and a little psychic; another gift I have which often came in handy when working with the elderly later on.

At the age of 15 months I started to walk but I cut my little toe on a nail which took a long time to heal and the infection spread across the rest of my toes. My mum took me to the baby clinic where it got treated although the doctors there said my foot looked like it had been scalded. I was allergic to cow's milk and other dairy products although I was weaned back onto it and over the years I have found though I can tolerate dairy to a degree.

When I was two years old my mother took me to have my ears pierced which was a painful and stressful experience. My mother recalls my ears were fine for at least six weeks until she replaced the earrings with gold studs. At this point my left ear went septic behind the lobe and my ear became a bit of a mess. The ear split and became infected and my ear took a long time to heal and the earrings had to be removed. The stress from the earrings could have triggered my first convulsion as apart from being a nervous child I was fine up until this point. It turned out I was allergic to gold, silver, nickel and many other metals which I have learned more about as the years have progressed. Neutropenia had not yet been considered or looked into.

I was two years old playing happily with my friends in the room next door when my mother heard a loud thudding sound. My mother came running into the room to find me squatting down jerking and foaming at the mouth. My eyes were rolling and I was making choking noises. Three months later I had another convulsion and I was taken to the children's hospital where they kept me in overnight for observation. At this point I was diagnosed with epilepsy and prescribed **Epilim™Syrup** medication and the full extent of my nervousness was exposed.

From then on, I was placed under a specialist and my life started to revolve around hospital visits, check-ups and GP appointments. In line with school I somehow had to find the balance between the side effects of the medication and my school work which became a constant battle. My mother became frustrated feeling that nothing was being achieved through the various hospital appointments and tests and the time my mother had to take off work in order to attend was also difficult. I myself struggled to keep up with my mother's stress and my own. Not that a child of my age was supposed to see or undergo such an experience. Let alone understand it.

I became afraid of my own shadow, loud noises, cars, bikes even going swimming or shopping with my mother put the fear of god into me. As a small child not even I understood or was able to communicate or explain to others what was going on inside my head. . I mentioned earlier that I had my first seizure when I was 2 years old and having had a number of convulsions I started taking Epilim™ syrup which caused many side effects as the years progressed. The syrup of course weakened my teeth and gums and eventually I was put onto Epilim™ tablets which I stayed on for many years or would return to periodically. Over the years I took many different types of medication though the three I remember taking up until the age of 15 were Epilim™, Tegretal™ and Kepra™. The medication was partly responsible for my neutropenia later in life. I was very self-aware but also highly attuned to my mother and as a result I took on a lot of my mother's stress though I found all this difficult to explain at the time, since being on medication had changed who I was. I later learned that many of the medication i took also caused anxiety and depression as a side effect.

Until I had my first convulsion I was a very intelligent child. I was very attractive, bubbly and confident until my first or second convulsion. Once I started taking Epilim™Syrup medication everything changed. I became frightened of noise and constantly sleepy. I became very withdrawn and isolated and found my school work difficult to manage since concentration was difficult. At around the age of five or six I suffered from a migraine and I was screaming. My mum called the doctor out. I was fine on this occasion although another convulsion followed shortly afterwards. I broke out in a sweat and developed red blotches on my skin all over my body. My mum called for an ambulance and I was taken to hospital where I was sedated and discharged the following morning.

Between the ages of two and seventeen my mother only ever recalls me having around ten seizures whilst on medication. My condition was well controlled as a child growing up; I found my epilepsy did not spiral out of control until I started my menstrual cycle. The control of my epilepsy allowed me to have greater independence although the main pitfall was the high dosage of medication which unfortunately affected my concentration and slowed down my learning ability.

My mother noticed that the brightness and intelligence I had demonstrated as a young child all changed once I started having seizures. My memory worsened as I got older and this had an effect on my spelling, punctuation and grammar. My short term memory, ability to remember my shopping list, phone numbers, names and faces was also affected.

The Epilim™Syrup may have worked for controlling my seizures however unbeknown to myself and anyone else, it was having a detrimental effect on the rest of my body. It was when I was out playing with friends and theyear that my second set of teeth were coming through when I learned just what effect the medication was having on my teeth and gums. As I turned a street corner I bumped into a friend of mine and my adult tooth came out from the root. It had landed just under my friend's eye and probably scared him for life! I did not know at that time we could have put the tooth back in using hot or warm milk.

After that my teeth and gums got worse. I was eight years old when the hospital diagnosed me with neutropenia (an abnormally low number of white blood cells) although at that point, the cause of the white cell deficiency was not known. I spent many years visiting the dental hospital until I was old enough to attend the adult dental surgery. Of course the dentist always blamed me for not looking after my teeth properly.

Due to having such a low birth weight, my skull was so tiny it affected my jaw, brain and blood. Being on medication from an early age made it difficult to know if medication was the only cause of my blood condition, the state of my gums and the metal allergies given the events of the first years of my life prior to the first convulsion.

I found my seizures easier to hide whilst at school because of the type of warning signs I experienced; and absence seizures were often mistaken for lack of concentration or daydreaming. As a result the many absence seizures I had were often never recorded or noted down. Epilim™ and Tegretal™ were the two main treatment methods I was given and while they worked well for seizure control, there were many unwelcome side effects which did not go unnoticed at school.

My mother's wish and dream for me was to be a popular child with lots of friends. In reality I was a loner with few friends and I spent most of my time on my own. I found school difficult although I enjoyed learning and attending school I found making friends of my own age challenging. I struggled to relate to people my own age and found small groups rather intimidating. I spent time with people my mother's age or older or would often spend time with children younger than myself which made me a suitable candidate for a babysitter as I became older; although by time I reached my teenage years looking after children became an issue due to my seizures.

The only company I had was my music and my books. I spent most of my time writing poetry or stories. I had the occasional friend from nursery and as the same group of school children all attended the same schools throughout, I grew up with the same crowd I met at nursery. It was a learning curve for me from a personal development point of view as I learned to overcome my fear and anxiety and improve my own self esteem.

The amount of medication I took made me sleepy, and as a result I had little interest in activities which was no doubt noticeable to anyone observing. I know how frustrating it can be for anyone caring for a child who is semi-conscious on medication and trying to get the child to catch up and be coherent, it is difficult. It is just as frustrating for the child who wants to play and be a normal child but is unable to do what everyone else is doing. Mum found that she too often felt a little restricted as to what she could and could not do, as she often felt ruled by social services. I was unable to go out without mum's fear of me having a seizure. I was unable to climb a wall or engage in various activities and I guess there was often a lot of anxiety about what I could and could not do which often left both me and my Mum feeling restricted. These restrictions did not go unnoticed by others which affected forming relationships both in and outside school. As a child I did not always understand this; I was often surrounded by fear. I dealt with this by surrounding myself with my own world. My anxiety was high and I was often frightened of my own shadow and as a result I spent a lot of time in my own room, I also had an invisible friend called Jenny, and she provided great company to a lonely child. I also enjoyed working with animals and as I grew up I had many pets.

Other children bullied and teased me through ignorance and stigma and while I enjoyed learning this turned school into something I hated.

Bullying took place for just about anything and not much was ever done about it in the school I attended. For example, I remember one girl inviting her friends round to her house and she came in school the next day upset. The children had picked on her because she did not have a wash basket and her dirty laundry was scattered about her bedroom.

In primary school the head teacher had a bed for me in his office and would often interrupt my younger brother every time I had a seizure. Obviously I was always concerned about the impact this had on my brothers education.

I can remember just how withdrawn I was as a child and how much the medication sent me to sleep. I found concentration in school rather difficult and I found it hard to make friends and socialise. Epilim™, Tegretal™ and Keppra™ controlled my seizures rather well though they carried a lot of side effects.

I recall how much the medication slowed my learning ability down. Everything I learned up to the age of four I basically forgot due to the effects of Epilim™. Epilim™ could also have been responsible for the decrease in my white cell count which has worsened over time. I was an intelligent child and very aware of my surroundings but the medication I took for my condition often set me back.

Keppra™ affected me in a way that I would walk into things like I was drunk and also falling over. The effect of Tegretal™ was difficult to identify because I had already been given my diagnoses of neutropenia and was visiting the dentist for all the problems I was having. I came out in rashes, had sore throats and bleeding gums. I seemed to have everything rolled into one so was unsure if Tegretal™ was benefitical for me. I chose to go back on Tegretal™ later on in my adult years but never felt I got any benefit from it or that it had any side effects.

I wasn't diagnosed with depression until after I left school and started studying at college, though I believe I was suffering from depression throughout my childhood long before I left school. The panic attacks never got mentioned until I started studying at college and doing my own research. It was then i also learned about anxiety.

Anxiety disorder was probably not recognised in children back then either, so I was labelled as "an emotional child". Not that anything ever changed over the years. I simply have a better understanding of myself and who I was in my earlier years. I used to experience terrible reoccurring dreams and nightmares that continued throughout school. I feel my dreams were caused by a combination of anxiety and seizures. No one picked up on how society's ignorance and lack of education could be a trigger for depression or how depression and anxiety could be linked or intertwined. The schools did nothing to educate children on stress or disability and so children were bullied for just about everything. I tried my best to keep to myself though it only made matters worse.

So I spent most of my time in doors locked away in my room listening to my music, reading or writing my diaries; and due to the difficulty with my concentration at school the teachers would give me extra help and support with my work. In primary school I was close to one friend who I lost contact with. I do recall we would spend a lot of our time on the grass hill in the school playground doing cartwheels on the grass although I did not like to participate too much for fear of causing a seizure. There were other children in the same year as me who would often ask me to play with them but I often refused to play out of shyness and fear that too much activity would trigger off my seizures. I would often be taken out of school and sit for hours with my mum to see a specialist at the hospital. I was ten years old and my care was split between two hospitals in Manchester. Although I did not mind going to one hospital. I hated been taken out of school for the long trip to the second. I not only had the long walk to the hospital but then the long wait for only a few minutes with the consultant; only to be told that anything I did could trigger a convulsion. These rules only added to my nerves and made me more anxious. I found that this was going to be a frustrating relationship I would have with the medical profession, throughout my life. As i got older i gained a better understanding and developed a better relationship with the many hospitals I encountered. There were some consultant appointments however in which I felt my meetings did actually achieve something, and teach me or help me in some way. They would benefit a lot in my future.

Back then however, I was angry with the hospitals and anyone who told me, **"You can't because of your epilepsy."** I hated the restrictions and the control and the fuss. All I wanted was to be free and able to have a simple and normal childhood.

There were a few occasions over the years where I was taken off medication and my concentration and focus returned which improved my social life at school and my ability to work. I was a different person of medication, I was happier and more alert.

I found myself being wrapped up in cotton wool and with a long list of rules and regulations of what I could and could not do which left me feeling rather restricted. I felt dizzy, angry and scared most of the time during my teenage years although I would often challenge myself to overcome my own fears and phobias. I found it difficult to understand my mother and could become very emotional over the slightest thing. However, as I got older I began to understand my mother's stress and frustration and why she was often upset. I found myself going through the same emotions that she had as I started to attend the hospital appointments by myself as I got older.

Chapter Two

An Angry Teenager

I left school **in 1994** at the age of fifteen with three GCSE'S and was seizure free for three years between the ages of sixteen and nineteen; although I recall the odd night time seizure and absence seizure. These slowly increased leading up to a tonic clonic seizure (**a type of generalised seizure affecting the entire brain**), that occurred in the kitchen when I was twenty years old. I never went to hospital and refused treatment until the age of twenty five.

My seizures were a lot easier to control as a child; I started out just having convulsions with a few absences, then they switched to night time seizures with a few tonic clonic seizures. As I grew older I had more absences and night time seizures with the occasional day time seizure which were known as **"fits"** back then. Once my menstrual cycle started I recall having partial seizures, absences and tonic clonics.

As a baby I slept a lot only waking for a feed, my tiredness and anxiety only deteriorated over the years not helped by medication and my seizures.

Everyone knew what a tonic clonic seizure was, which people still call a "grand mal" today; although trying to explain absence seizures, complex partial seizures or any other type of seizure to my school friends or teachers was hard work. Mum recalls my night time seizures but because she had rarely seen my absences or partials she does not recall them. I regularly received a range of diagnoses from the hospitals over the years which only added to mine and my mother's anxiety. I can recall having practically every seizure listed apart from the photo sensitive epilepsy and status.

In terms of hospital treatment, over the years there were many arguments over what type of epilepsy I had, or whether it was non-epileptic attack disorder **(NEAD)**.Were they fits or seizures, **syncope** (fainting attacks) or drug resistance epilepsy? Due to the complexity of my condition including migraine attacks, epilepsy and fainting attacks; and the symptoms for all three conditions being very similar I found separating my symptoms and knowing which condition was responsible for them very difficult. Often EEG scans were normal and as I could get warnings with both my migraines and seizures as a teenager I was never quite sure if I actually had epilepsy. I still suffer migraine attacks today and often my migraine attacks can be the result of a seizure and stress.

I find I get migraines as a result of the weather, after spending too long using the computer or even watching TV. I used to get migraine attacks during my menstrual cycle and often I could experience a migraine without having had a seizure. My migraine could simply be a warning that a small seizure had occurred in the brain. I was never quite sure which of my symptoms had been triggered by my epilepsy and which were non-epilepsy related. Therefore I could see why so many of the consultants were confused. At the age of fifteen however, I was still struggling to understand myself and getting rather frustrated with the various diagnoses I was been given.

I was not the only one who had questions. Every consultant I came into contact with also had questions. Until someone could give me the answers I chose to go my own way.

At the age of 15 years old I decided to stop attending the hospital and come off my medication because of the difficult relationship I had with various consultants and doctors. I was at that rebellious age and felt that the medication slowed me down. I wanted the opportunity to live my life like the rest of the world without restrictions. I never had a learning disability or mental health condition, it was the medication that affected my development and sent me to sleep and there were many occasions when I was asked if I would be better off at a special needs school. I never felt this was necessary there was nothing special about me. I grew up with people I knew who attended the same high school and I would take whatever ignorance they presented to me. Instead, the school gave me a support worker to assist me during my first year after which I was placed in all the lowest sets. Given how well I did in college I never quite understood why I was ranked so low.

I wasn't diagnosed with dyslexia until I was investigated for neuro-surgery **in 2009**. I feel that if I had been assessed for dyslexia earlier I would have progressed further in subjects like English and maths. I enjoyed drama and arts and found I did well in these subjects. I gained my RSA One and Two and got merits and distinctions in both despite struggling in English. I left school with good GCSE's and did well in college finally graduating with Scottish qualifications.

I experienced a level of bullying in high school that I felt was born of ignorance and as I was an emotional person and afraid of my own shadow, I was too afraid to stick up for myself because it was drummed into me that if I did this it could bring on a seizure. I took a few years of this kind of stick before I finally snapped and started to defend myself. I found things changed after that, I started to get punished by the teachers for fighting instead. I had friends in school and learned various life skills and social skills. I guess this gave me some degree of confidence whilst in school.

I found it easier if I did not mention my condition. I was also having complex partial seizures that were pre-ceded by warning signs; so my epilepsy was easier to hide. Concentration was easier without medication and making friends and finding acceptance was also easier if I kept my condition quiet. There was still so much stigma and discrimination around, and I learned that by keeping quiet about my epilepsy, I would progress further.

After leaving school, I started work and took a few years off from the hospital, only visiting my GP on occasion for counselling or advice, or if I needed medication for a condition I could not treat myself.

It was in this same year that I was also introduced to my father through a cousin of mine. Epilepsy ran in my father's side of the family and I was keen to learn more about my father and if my epilepsy had been inherited. I knew a little bit about him and his side of the family from my mother and a few of my cousins that had attended the same school.

My cousin who was in the year above me in high school arranged the meeting between me and my father. I was a wash of mixed emotions, and making the phone call was about the most nerve wracking moment of all.

I could not wait to meet up with my Father outside my favourite restaurant. I recall feeling a little disappointed when my father picked me up in his car and took me to *his* favourite eating place instead. I was so nervous at the time I simply picked at my food. However, I felt complete, having finally met my father after only ever being told about him. I always used to send my dad Father's Day cards and then upset myself that I never heard anything back.

I wanted to share the strain of the stress I had been experiencing for all those years and I had visions of my father assisting and supporting me throughout the rest of my journey. However it was not meant to be. The reality was that my father did not wish to have the responsibility of all my stress or even share any of what my mother had been through. He was not as mature as I had imagined him to be. On our first meeting my father criticised me and pulled me down which looking back, I now feel only contributed to my anxiety and depression. I realised from then on I had expected too much that I was not going to get the love and attention from my father that I had craved for all those years.

At the same time I was also introduced to some new siblings. My father had re-married on more than one occasion and as a result I had two new sisters and two new brothers, one of which was not that much younger than myself. Although I spent some time with each of them we never really got along, and even though we would be introduced to each other once again through the internet. I found that I did not feel part of this new family that I had discovered.

When I was fifteen, I also started a Y.T.S course in the hope that I could get some work experience in some kind of caring capacity, before I attended college. I did not tell my employers or the trainers about my medical condition. Following the meeting with my father my emotions were all over the place and I found I was struggling to concentrate on the course. I was suffering from depression and anxiety which did not go down too well in the work placement, which was at a residential care home.

In addition to feeling so unhappy, I was left to do a lot of the work on my own, I did not yet feel ready for so much responsibility. I found myself having many arguments with the matron and trainers at the college, and after a harsh exchange of words I was thrown out.

A few months later I signed up at college, feeling isolated, anxious and lonely. I was starting to miss my friends from high school and very much in need of some company.

I decided to re-take my exams and continue my training course but this time through a college GNVQ, and being around my friends helped me. I enjoyed working in care but under the Y.T.S scheme I was under too much stress. I still carried a lot of resentment towards the hospital and felt restricted as to what I could and could not do; so whilst studying at college, I found myself rebelling in a lot of ways. It was my way of finding out who I was and doing some self-development.

In 1996, at the age of seventeen I decided I wanted to have a go at driving lessons much to my GP's horror. It is actually illegal to drive if you have uncontrolled epilepsy.

Of course he wrote in his GP notes the contradictions of having epilepsy and the laws, rules and regulations **according to the DVLA**. Even so I was undeterred and applied for my provisional licence, missing out the minor detail of my medical history and a provisional licence was received. My granddad gave me a copy of the theory test to study and I booked myself in for some lessons. My GP then informed me that in order to meet DVLA requirements I would have to start back on medication. So I put in a request to see my GP notes to assist with my memory and I kept a diary of my seizures over the years. When I looked at my doctor's notes, my GP had indicated that I had *asked* to go back on medication. This I knew I did *not* request due to the symptoms or side effects of the medication. However since I would be unable to have driving lessons without my medication, **in 1997** I reluctantly went back on medication for a period of two years in order to learn to drive.

I was due to start my health and social care course at college as I was planning to work with the elderly once I had completed the course and thought I would improve my career prospects if I could drive.

I knew Epilim™ and Tegretal™ controlled my seizures well as a child but had no idea if they would work as an adult. Going back on medication once again made me withdrawn and I struggled with my course work and found working in a care capacity difficult. Having driving lessons was also difficult. I went through three different driving instructors and several months went by without having a lesson. I never did get past my theory test. My mother seems to think I was scaring the driving instructors off with my seizures.

I eventually left work after the deaths of residents and because the hours I was working had started to affect my depression and cause me to feel more withdrawn and stressed. Neither did it help my seizures. The symptoms of anxiety remained with me and in **1998** I began studying other courses in order to reduce this. Although the courses helped I would often find myself surrounded by a vicious circle. This was especially the case, at the time of my menstrual cycle. I would start with one seizure, followed by a cluster which would continue with feelings of anxiety and depression. My employers would often tell me to have some time off work, thinking or assuming that I would be ok after a few days. Even though doctors prescribed the contraceptive pill when I was fifteen years old to regulate my periods I found this never really helped.

Quite often when I returned to work, I would still experience the occasional seizure, fainting attack or even simply tiredness and fatigue. I noticed how my seizures affected my concentration and how the attitude of my work colleagues changed towards me.

I found myself out of work on several occasions and by **the year 2000** I was diagnosed with anxiety and panic attacks. I often attended therapy in order to learn to control my anxiety and depression however this only ever worked on a short term basis. I found studying, researching and personal development courses helpful as they gave me greater understanding of myself and others. I also ditched my father and decided not to bother with his side of the family as it was doing my emotional wellbeing no good. I finished off my courses, gave up work and decided to focus on my own personal development. **In 2000** I did my Reiki One followed by my Reiki Two a year later.

I found it therapeutic to practice Reiki and meditation. Not only was the Reiki helping my seizures but I found it was also helpful for my anxiety.

In 2001 I decided to leave Salford; I had been wrapped up in cotton wool for far too long. I was now in my early twenties and still lived at home. I had only just learned how to cook and had never really been out of the city without my mum by my side. I had found friends on the estate I now lived on but I was starting to get bored.

Mum had decided to buy a caravan in Cumbria so that she could be closer to her new job. It was not until my mum had passed her driving test that I too found my own independence. Until that point I was a rather shy person and quite introvert, I had always been emotional. It was now time to find myself and improve my confidence. As I walked away from my family, there was just me and my mum. As much as we were close it was now time to break away from her apron strings. This time though it was my mother who was following me.

Though I considered myself a risk taker and a sociable person, despite my epilepsy, I was often perceived as a little naive. Since leaving school I had many jobs. I had gained many qualifications and even made more friends, although I was still a loner. Mum was now working away and only coming home for the occasional weekend. I was no longer working and spent my time walking the dog and helping out a neighbour. When my mother came home one weekend and told me she had bought a caravan I seized the opportunity to spread my wings and seek my independence.

38

I had found a college up in Scotland, but did not tell my mum at that point in time. She thought she was taking me somewhere local. As I sat there in the car watching mum check round one last time to make sure we had everything and take one last look at the house, I wondered if mum had any concerns about leaving town.

The area had way too many bad memories for us, although we knew the area and the people well. It was the stress of hospital visits, the stigma of living with epilepsy and the emotional effects that I wanted to escape from. Most of the people we knew all grew up with us and I knew some of the younger adults from school. There were too many memories, and not ones that mum or I wished to remember.

"So, are we ready for our next adventure?" Mum asked, as we drove out of the close. "Yep!" I replied, watching the families come out of their houses to watch us drive off. Of course I never knew that in the next century there would be internet sites and social media that would bring such people back from the past or how such internet sites would have an influence on my life.

Once we were on the motorway I realised I still hadn't told my mum where it was that I was going.

"Which direction?" Mum asked as we jumped on to the M61 heading in the wrong direction.

"Oops we have to turn round mum, I'm heading up north, and we might even be able to stay at your place tonight?" I replied.

"Why are we going that far?" She asked with a look of surprised shock on her face. I glanced at the dog wondering how he would react to his new surroundings, he had never lived in the countryside before; he had lived in the city or spent most of his life on housing or council estates ever since he was a pup.

"Err yeah mum, I've got a residence in Edinburgh." I announced.

Turning the car around as soon as we reached an exit, mum looked at me with shock still on her face. "You kept that quiet, and why didn't you tell me?"

"Err, I was not sure how to tell you mum." The truth was that I was still too afraid to communicate with my mother. I learned more about my stress and anxiety as the years progressed but for now it was all about improving my confidence.

Though mum and I are very close, sometimes we are more like sisters, we have this love hate relationship. Sometimes this closeness can often be the reason why I have difficulty expressing myself or even talking to my mum at times, even something like telling my mum I am moving to Scotland. I find myself leaving it until the last minute. I mean mum did not tell me she was giving up the house when she started working in Cumbria; she just came home one day and announced it like it was some promotion.

If I had told my mum when I first started looking at courses and colleges in Scotland then I feared my mum might talk me out of it. I knew my mum suffered some kind of anxiety disorder herself although she had little understanding of her own condition, and my mother had always been over protective. I was the eldest of her children, my brother being three years younger than me, and healthy.

My mum was also at a very young age herself when she had me, and having epilepsy I guess in her eyes I am still her little girl. My mum just wanted the best for me; although at times being over protective of your child can only make things worse for them when they are growing up. I had no idea mum was already thinking of moving in that direction anyway. I know the two of us have always been so close we are almost telepathic but to both be making such huge plans within months of one another showed how much we were on the same level and was amazing. I mean, my mum must have been looking at caravans in Cumbria while I was looking at colleges and courses. I knew we were spiritually connected from a very early age. My first premonition was when I was six years old, when my grandmother took me with her to a cleaning job. I had never been to the town before but I described the building before we arrived. I do not have that many memories from my early childhood though when I had conversations with my mother and grandmother I would often describe events that took place that both women swore they had never spoken about before. I often felt like I was my mother's guide and vice versa. We would both go out to the shops separately and come back with the same items even though we never went to the same shops. It was as though we were reading each other's mind. Over the years if my mother sensed I was in danger she would often ring me up or vice versa which often stopped or prevented me from getting into many scrapes or accidents from occurring.

However, despite this closeness my mum has always wanted her freedom to go her own way yet at the same time I knew she would always worry about me. Over the years she had me wrapped up in cotton wool. I wanted to break away from this at the first opportunity I got and mum moving to Cumbria was this opportunity. I could show her just how independent I was. I know parents have a tendency to still perceive their children as teenagers even when they have passed a certain age. Or they continue to see their children as children even into adulthood, and it must be harder to let go when a child has an illness or medical condition. I have always faced this battle with my mum and though sometimes I felt I needed her by my side, at times finding the right balance became overwhelming.

I have memories of walking to hospital appointments and my mother always being angry. Though I understand now that my mother was dealing with her own demons, it took some time and a lot of research to understand that anxiety and mental health runs in my mother's side of the family. I was never quite sure back then why mum was always angry, and this made me fearful, although now I understand, seeing the frustration other mothers experience with their own children.

As I grew older and started to challenge the doctors and various consultants myself, I started to understand my mother's frustration. I learned that my mother was never angry with *me* although it often felt that way. As I started to experience the same frustration that she had, I too started to challenge the system and my own relationship with my mother began to improve.

A lot of the people who lived around me knew me from school and I found I was unable to move on whilst living in the same area due to the large amount of stigma and assumptions that surrounded me. It was a tough neighbourhood and I was not a tough person. There were plenty of people that I knew who were often getting involved with the police and my brother often mixed with those crowds. I found myself dodging certain people on the way home just for some peace.

Mum tried her best to keep the peace, however I guess when parents get involved in children's squabbles sometimes that only makes the situation worse even though the parents get involved out of love and concern. That is not always for the best. I knew I had to get involved more and look at my experiences from a different point of view or perspective, which is not always easy when you are caught up in all the pain and hurt or living in a society where you are meant to stick up for yourself.

My mum would often come home to her car smashed up or windows broken or phone calls from the police which did not help her relationship with the neighbours. Eventually my brother went to live with his grandparents and we moved again to another estate which was no better.

I guess this was the reason why in the end both me and mum moved away, too many memories and a past that neither one of us wanted to be connected with anymore, haunted us. I had to move on in order to deal with my anxiety and find myself.

When a person is so full of resentment and negativity, trying to change who you are is very difficult until they remove themselves from their situation and look at it again possibly from a third persons perspective. Scotland was a new and exciting experience for me as it was a new start. At the same time I was not sure if I was excited or apprehensive about my new experience.

"So how long does it take to get to Scotland mum?" I asked now she was on the right junction.

"We will have to stop at a garage and fill up with petrol I'm not sure we have enough for Scotland."

Chapter Three

The Halls

Upon arriving in Scotland mum found herself driving around in circles, I guess she was not used to one way systems, or not like this one anyway. In the end we had to stop and ask some local fire fighters who were parked up with their fire engine where the local college was, not realising we were on the other side of town.

Eventually we found the college on what looked like a countryside road. I was surprised, I thought Edinburgh was a city, yet here we were driving down narrow country lanes towards what looked like a large manor house.

Inside the building, I felt like I had just walked into a boarding school or a countryside hotel. A woman approached me and she seemed to know who I was, and after introducing herself she took me to a table where I paid my deposit for the halls of residence and she informed me that I would be studying and staying at the same place. The woman gave me a map showing me where I needed to go before sending us on our way.

The halls of residence were busy with activity. I was told the girls would reside on one side of the building and the boys would remain on the other, we could mix and enter each other's quarters until a certain time then both would have to go back to their own quarters. I suddenly felt like I was back at school with all these rules. There was a kitchen and shower room which was shared, a communal area and laundry room. Very different from living at home with my mum, now I had to get used to reporting in and out of the building, sharing facilities with others and living next door to a lot more noise than I was used to. This was not only the start of my new adventure but also my freedom, and I was excited.

Having settled in and locked my room, mum checked the car before we took a tour around the rest of the building. We met some of my teachers and I checked out the restaurant, swimming pool and gym. The local B&B was just off site and the pubs were just up the road.   We took a short walk to the local shopping centre; and then mum checked I was ok for money before leaving me to my own fate.

I was now an independent person for the first time in my life aged just twenty-three and with no idea what I was letting myself in for. It was the furthest distance away from home that I had ever been in my entire life, other than when I went on holiday to America with a friend from school for my eighteenth birthday. There were many other times when me and my friend went on holiday together but often we went on holiday with her parents.   Going to America was the first time I was away without my mother and this had given me my first taste of independence.

Back in the halls of residence, I sat on my bed looking out the window, with no idea where to put my belongings. So far I had only a suitcase, kettle, CD player and CDs, posters, some of my own bedding, a few towels, my clothes, a few books and a few things I needed for college which included stationery. Mum said she would bring things up to me as she visited; the idea was that I would make a note of what I needed and then provide her with a list.   The rest of my things from home would go into storage. When I found my own place, then I would call for them. Right now though, I was starting with just my suitcase and a few extras.

This was a new adventure for me, I had officially left home! At the time I was too excited about my new life to be aware of my anxiety or my seizures. I had successfully found a place to live and a college course and planned to find a job, so I was not thinking about the different ways in which stress and anxiety can affect a person subconsciously or without a person being aware of a medical condition. As far as I was concerned, I had a fresh start. I had forgotten about my mother, my old life back in Manchester and Salford and even any stress that might have occurred. What I did not know is just how quickly my old life could come back to haunt me.

I had a lot of personal development to do and I would embark on some of that work during my college course; however subconsciously my anxiety was still present and physical symptoms were making themselves known although I was not sure why. At the time I was unaware that what I was experiencing were symptoms of anxiety. I assumed they were symptoms of excitement or overwhelming tiredness due to the adjustment period, as at that time I was not home sick.

Over the next few months I made friends and settled in to the course I had enrolled on. I found a job working at the rail station behind the bar and even made friends with some of the locals. My confidence began to improve living in the city and I even started to pick up the accent. Work plays an important part in helping a person improve their confidence. So to take that away from a person is not only going to be a dent in a person's personal development but it isolates a person further. With a medical condition like epilepsy then socially work is very important to a person's mental health. Epilepsy is isolating enough so for me work has always been my life line. I have found that socialising and working has always helped me feel like an equal person and made me feel useful.

However despite how well I got on in the city of Edinburgh and just how much I was enjoying living there, there was something haunting me, something from my past was creeping up when I just wanted to forget about it. I thought that perhaps no one here would notice and just maybe I could leave my past behind.

Time passed quickly and mum came up whenever she got the chance, bringing up more of my things with each visit. However I never told her about the part of my life that kept haunting me, I did not want to worry her I was an independent woman now.

One day while at work I was asked to manage the café. Brilliant! I was not only working behind the bar and in the kitchen but I was now managing the café for them too. I loved my job in the rail station. I did not mind the long shifts or coming back home smelling of stale booze and cigarettes and I found I had a good social life at the station. I never really took much notice of the financial cost of having such independence as I was having too much of a good time. After work I would often go out with the staff and mix with the customers. I found everyone who worked at the rail station to be rather friendly and I got to know shop owners and customers working on the high street within the first few months. Working and living in Edinburgh was nothing like my life in the North West of England. Here, I felt that my epilepsy was never an issue and settling in to life and work was easy. However, there were a few down sides to living in Scotland's capital.

Edinburgh was very expensive and I knew once I finished my course I would be unable to continue to fund my lifestyle. Some nights after work we would all go out with the staff to the clubs and pubs, or I would sit in the pubs in Rose Street with some of the locals or staff from the station. I was only working shifts and sometimes the part time hours didn't cover my rent let alone the social life I so wanted and needed. I was unable to cover the bank loan and over draft and found myself starting to struggle. My mum was constantly coming up to check on me and I often resented her help as much as I needed it. I admired my own independence and wanted to show everyone just how independent I could be.

I never wanted my job at the rail station to end and was fearful that if they ever found out about my epilepsy they might sack me. I was now managing the café, supervising the bar and was very much my own boss in the kitchen. My hours had increased and I was now technically working two jobs and as a result I found that the stress levels were starting to have an effect. One particular day when I was managing the café became a day of judgement for me. I was doing the stock take in the café while the place was quiet, with not that many customers as we were waiting for the next train load to arrive before the café got busy. The next thing I knew there was a security guard who was also a first aider sitting with me.

"Are you ok do you need a glass of water? Are you hurt anywhere?" He asked.

"Eh??" What was he fussing over? I was confused, with no idea who he was or what he was going on about?

"Don't worry hen," he said "your boss is on her way then you can come with me fill in some forms".

Slowly I came round and it suddenly dawned on me what had happened. It was clear looking at where I had been standing that I had experienced a seizure and sat or leant myself on the dishwasher and burnt my back or there about anyway. Only I had no warning that the seizure was coming on nor did I feel any different on that particular day. "Oh damn" I thought. "What will happen now?"

I had successfully started a new course, relocated and found employment. Well so much for the new start…

My boss and the customers were different in their attitude, compared to what I was used to. They were very supportive and it didn't seem to bother them that I had kept this a secret. My boss took over while I went with the first aid assistant and filled in the forms. When I was ready I went back to the café and approached my manager. She simply asked me if there was any chance of it happening again on that day, and whether I would be able to finish my shift, and with that she left me to it leaving me in shock.

I finished my shift with no problems and without any further incident. For me that goes to show that there is not always a need for an ambulance to be called out and for the person with epilepsy who has had the seizure to be taken away from their job role.

I had many accidents whilst working at the rail station and not all of them were down to my epilepsy or required a trip to hospital and I remained at the rail station until I eventually moved to Glasgow. I also took on a second job for extra cash as a support worker working night shifts for an adult with mental health problems.

I found Scotland had a whole different attitude towards my medical condition which pleased me and helped my personal development and confidence a great deal. I also made quite a few friends and enrolled on a few personal development courses that complimented my HNC course. I also found Scotland to be full of creative people and I felt very much at home during my time there. To be honest I did not want to leave and probably would never have left Scotland if it was not for the way my path turned out.

Back at the halls I thought I had better come clean with the staff and some of my new friends, about my condition; perhaps it would be better to mention it, as I had no intention at this stage of going back on my medication or even going back to the hospital.

Chapter Four

Moving on

Unfortunately, the halls worked out as a temporary arrangement. When we broke up from college for the Christmas holidays the halls chucked us out so we all had to go home which meant packing up and leaving our jobs.

Therefore I was forced to take two weeks leave from my job at the rail station while I searched for a more permanent arrangement.

Luckily I did not have to move far, I found a place just up the road from where I was studying. A woman was renting out her spare room which worked well for me and it was not that much more than I was paying at the halls. Obviously it meant leaving my friends at the halls but I wanted to concentrate on my studies anyway. This would be my second move since leaving mum, my first flat share and first experience of living with a stranger. My landlord was really nice, a private woman from Ireland, and not much older than me. I gathered that she was self-employed and a very successful person. With me spending most of my time at college and work I guessed that we would hardly see much of each other anyway. Musselburgh was a nice village and one of the girls from my course had a house just up the road from where I was living so I hoped to see more of her. I liked the people on my course, however our group ended up being one of the smallest. At times, this was a good thing as we worked well as a small group. At other times I wondered if it would have been better to double up with one of the other courses.

In a way meeting my landlord was one of the best moves I ever made in terms of my personal development. It was through her that was I introduced to another course that helped me to do something that I have mentioned earlier. I was able to look at my past from a third party perspective and move forward. I also met some interesting people and made some good friends who I am still in touch with today.

I am a strong believer in the fact that things happen for a reason. Like I was meant to move to Scotland, I was meant to have the experiences I had, even though some may not have worked out in the way I would have liked. I was only living at Musselburgh for about ten months before I moved out back up the road just around the corner from the college.

By then I had lost contact with my friends from the halls. I hardly saw the girl from the Scottish borders now that she worked more hours at the cinema and I had no idea where she was living or if she had been accepted on the University Degree course. As for my other friends from the Shetland Islands I did not know whether they had gone back home.

Since the seizure in the café I had many more in the pub, and I think the customers were starting to notice. One customer in particular seized her opportunity to take advantage, and tried to steal my identity. It was at this point; when she was confronted that I realised just how much people think they can take advantage of someone with epilepsy. When the girl was confronted about her deception, I had quite a few pint glasses in my hands. It was a scary moment as I thought she was going to hit me and I might have the glasses chucked in my face. I knew then that I needed to leave my job, as even though the girl was barred from the pub, I did not feel safe afterwards.

I concentrated on working full time as a support worker, closer to where I was living. This time I found a job that matched my qualifications and this job allowed me to be my own boss with more hours and more money. I only had a few months left on my course and soon would be graduating so the money would come in handy as I was hoping to do a diploma or a psychotherapy degree course next, over in Glasgow.

The new job had extra responsibility and at this point I was still having difficulty confronting my condition which remained to be a big deal, as although I was able to look at my epilepsy from a different perspective, I still resented myself. At least I still carried no resentment for anyone else or the country I was born and grew up in. I was getting there slowly, I just needed more time that was all.

I still had many unanswered questions; such as that old argument about whether or not my condition was epilepsy or was it something else? And did I want a proper investigation to address this before I was willing to accept it? Did I want some proper evidence before I went back on the drugs, since I had seen and felt what the drugs did to a person?

There was of course the added stress and anxiety disorder which often got in the way of my diagnoses. I found I often took on board my mother's stress and anxiety which meant work and what other people said could affect me deeply. Often how people treated me whenever I had seizures affected my depression and I could enter a vicious circle. I found most of this very emotional. I studied a lot of personal development courses whilst in Scotland and enhanced my counselling training with holistic therapy and extra add on training. I found not only did this help with my own personal development but with my education too. I was becoming more assertive and much stronger but still found my anxiety disorder to be a challenge. With my anxiety and epilepsy combined I still found it difficult to distinguish which condition I was experiencing. So work often became a problem for me.

Trying to get someone who has never had epilepsy or experience of taking the medication to understand what it is like being drugged up is extremely difficult. Getting this message across to others would be challenging, especially when someone like myself found it difficult to adapt to life and a world that others took for granted. I understand just how frustrating it is for a parent or carer trying to get someone who is drugged up to cooperate on a day to day basis. However, most employers, friends and work colleagues have no idea. If I was to get on in life, and live my life like everyone else I knew I had a better chance if I stayed off the medication; but it was a choice between controlling the seizures or staying off the medication and risking my condition spiralling out control.

The courses I enrolled on helped my personal development a great deal and had the added benefit of meeting lots of people from the classes I joined. I felt I progressed further during the time I spent in Edinburgh than I did during all the years I lived in Manchester. The problem was I was spending money like it was going out of fashion. Many of the courses I enrolled on were private and expensive.

As I had not lived in Scotland long I was only able to apply for funding for one course so I had to use my savings to pay for the rest. The new flat was a three bedroom property on a small close, owned by an African family whose daughter still lived there; the other two rooms were rented out. One to myself and the other to a lad from Glasgow. The three of us got on well and occasionally the girl's family would come over and we would all have tea together.

I am not entirely sure what course the girl was studying but the guy we shared with was studying to be an actor. Other than a role in an advertisement for the Edinburgh to Glasgow train I am not sure if he had any other TV work while we were sharing accommodation. He moved back to Glasgow so we lost touch; however if he does ever pick up this book I would love to know what he is doing now and if he ever made it. I met a few actors whilst living in Edinburgh and most of them had seasonal work during the Edinburgh festival.

There was so much to do in Edinburgh, I never got bored of the beach, the city or even just jumping on the bus and going for a wander in a new part of town, or checking out a village. I found so much inspiration for my poems whilst living in Edinburgh. However as I enjoyed the expensive life money soon started to run dry.

I never did quite get the hang of saving up while I was in Scotland. I guess I was just too busy enjoying myself; I had so many dreams and ambitions. One of these was to start my own business once I qualified as a psychotherapist and the other was to publish my poetry.

Of course while I was working and living the high life there was little chance in publishing my book. I went on to discover that sadly no one seemed to care about poetry anymore; if I was to publish my work I would have to pay for the privilege and there was no way I could afford that.

I had already approached several publishers and magazines none of which were interested. Some were nice enough to send my work back with hints and help on how to present my work. Others sent me letters informing me about copyright and the cost of publication and as such it would be another four or five years before I would get my first book published. I found many publishers but all they gave me were hints and tips rather than the opportunity that I really wanted.

Eventually I graduated from college. On the day of my graduation my mum invited my aunt, uncle and my cousin to come up for the event. They all stayed at the local B&B next door to the college I was attending. We had a true Scottish graduation with bagpipes and a seminar. I even wore the graduation gown and received a scroll. Of course my mum scoffed at my choice of clothing as I selected a brown outfit rather than traditional black trousers and white blouse. Not that I minded, it was an event I wanted to remember and I have never been the type of person to conform.

The gentleman playing the bagpipes gave me a piece of advice and perhaps I should have taken this on; however if I had then I might not have had the experiences I had subsequently, leading to future events. Those experiences were what led to me to write this book. I had made quite a few friends and learned a lot about myself through my experiences at the rail station and the library, and this had made me rethink just how relaxed and comfortable I was getting. I had done a lot of self-awareness work and discovered more about my spiritual self and this helped me to confront my epilepsy although I still wanted to push my medical condition to one side. As much as I loved Edinburgh and would have preferred to stay, I no longer felt secure since I had my identity stolen by the woman at the station and a guy stealing my bag at the library. I felt it was time to move on, although I was not yet ready to go home. Perhaps the two events were necessary to make me aware of just how much I was letting my guard down. In addition my money was running low. I had a choice of applying for university in Edinburgh or moving to Glasgow. At the same time I also felt home sick although I was unsure who or what I was homesick for.

Destiny has a funny way of revealing its self. I guess we all have our destiny set out before us however the journey through life and the various paths we take can be based on the choices we make which can affect the length of time it takes us to reach our destiny. Does that mean I should have taken the guy in the kilt up on his advice or continued to push my determination a little further?

"Don't go no further," he said. "You have done enough lass, you have all the qualifications you need. It's time to move on and go home hen."

My mum agreed with him and taking me aside she asked me what I wanted to do now. I told her that I had the option of going to university and staying in Edinburgh or moving to Glasgow where I already had been accepted on a different course taking me in a new direction. There, I also had a place to stay where the guy who owned the college also owned a house in a little town just outside Glasgow. I had already been over there and met my tutor, seen the house and had a look round the college. This place was different again, he taught in a house outside the city of Glasgow, and his house where I would be living was huge. My ego just wanted to stay in Scotland a bit longer although my intuition was telling me this set up probably would not work.

However, I was not prepared to tell my mum that, so I stopped listening to reason and my determination once again took over. I knew I had to start again by finding another job, I was low on funds and as the course in Glasgow was a privately funded course I wouldn't be able to get funding for it. However I would keep that anxiety to myself; I didn't want to worry my mum; she now had her own life and I wanted to prove to her that I could make a go of it up here in the north. So after the graduation ceremony when we went for a meal I told the family all about my plans for new adventures in Glasgow and that maybe at the next graduation they could check Glasgow out.

Moving to Glasgow was an experience on its own and nothing like Edinburgh. In terms of my development, moving to Glasgow taught me a few more lessons one of which was that skeletons and secrets have a funny way of revealing themselves. I have learned that I cannot hide from my own skeletons and secrets no matter how far away I move. At the same time my journey made me a stronger person, my confidence improved and I was able to bring my experience to my future campaigns. Up until I moved to Scotland I was constantly wrapped up in cotton wool so I needed to break away to show people that I was a capable adult.

Chapter Five

Glasgow

The house in Glasgow was nothing like I expected. There were only two other people sharing the place. We had a downstairs shower and toilet, an upstairs bathroom and in each of the rooms we had our own sink. There were at least six bedrooms upstairs, and at least three more downstairs and the kitchen was a decent size. We had a communal living room and dining room and a huge driveway. Outside there was a very large garden –I'm sure we could have got lost in it if any of us had dared to go for a walk.

The area I was staying in was more like a village than a town. We had a few restaurants, shops, cafes and pubs and could walk to the nearest large supermarket or nearest town which, if you were feeling fit and healthy, would take around half an hour to reach. There was a bus that would take you into the city and various other towns and local shopping centres although it was sometimes easier to get the trains and underground to commute.

Glasgow had two rail stations and a bus station so I was never stuck for choice. It was pretty easy for me to get to college although on the odd weekend I would have to get a taxi unless I got a lift in as with most places in Glasgow it was a case of getting a bus or train into the city and then a second form of transport back out again unless you knew where you were going. I never did get the hang of transport or travel around the city. I still get lost to this day which might explain why Glasgow never did work out for me. Unlike most people I chose to stay local, working in the pubs in the area where I was staying. When that didn't work out I got a part time job in a local shopping centre just a few stops from my accommodation. Unlike Edinburgh I was afraid to venture too far from my accommodation, however I did check out the cost of local accommodation just down the road from the course I was enrolled on. The area did not look particularly safe however, so I chose to stay put. I liked where I was working and I liked where I was living. During the day I would venture a little further and meet up with friends, though I often found myself back on familiar ground. How I missed Edinburgh, unfortunately I did not have the cash to move back otherwise I would have done.

Soon I started to become home sick though I was unsure what or where I was pining for exactly. Was I missing Edinburgh or England? Was I missing my mum or my old life in Manchester? Either way it was clear my life in Glasgow was not going as I had planned. I had completed the first year of the advanced diploma course; although the goal post had been changed and I was looking at completing three years in order to gain the whole degree. It was clear I could not afford it without taking some time out to work full time and raise some funds. My business venture was not working out since I had insufficient money to commute and my new job in the shopping centre was only part time and did not pay well enough. I found myself spending more and more time in bed, lacking in motivation and enthusiasm. I struggled to find the links and contacts I needed for my business and course to succeed and had little energy to go out and socialise or even *try* to make Glasgow work for me.

I still needed somehow to gain experience for my course and I had to find a way to pay for this. I got a voluntary post working with Victim Support which gave me some experience in the High Court however this was still not enough, so I went on a Small Business Gateway course to get some advice and help with my business plan.

I knew that setting up my own business was going to be a difficult one in Glasgow, but nevertheless, I thought my experience working with the homeless, doing counselling courses, graduating and working in the courts would be enough. I had a few offers of running groups in various locations around Glasgow; however they were only test runs and having met up with these people and being interviewed I was turned down for not having life experience, despite running the courses for free and paying for all the costs myself. The odd group I did manage to run unfortunately was not enough to secure me a contract. I was not sure what I was doing wrong according to small business gateway I had a good business plan, done some good work and had a lot of experience and good qualifications. I had obtained references, done all the relevant training; including epilepsy awareness training through a charity I supported, my basic first aid training and challenging behaviour training.

It was not until later on when I moved back to Manchester and started my own research (together with chairing a support group in Salford for adults and families living with epilepsy; becoming involved in voluntary work and campaigns for several charities), that I realised it had been my epilepsy that had been getting in the way of running my own business up in Scotland. I found myself sleeping more than I was being active. I had friends up in Scotland but I started to see less of them. Relationships were not working out and although I had a boyfriend I found I no longer had the motivation to continue with the relationship. I wanted to go home but I was no longer sure where home was. Slowly the house mates started leaving the big house I was living in and I found myself feeling isolated and lonely.

One event I can recall happened when my house mate from Australia threw a house party and had some friends stay over. I am not sure if it was the alcohol or if it just happened to be my time of the month or I was just unlucky. Up until then I had managed to hide my epilepsy from my friends in Glasgow. I remember feeling my attack coming on this time; and when I came round there were a few people sitting with me and it appeared that I had spilt my drink on the carpet.

I ended up spending the night talking about epilepsy and my medical history. After which my landlord heard about it and I ended up bringing up the subject during a therapy session with him. After that I seemed to do a lot of talking and thinking, not just in the house but at work in the shop, the pubs the workshops, while at the dentist, whilst at college and out with friends. I was having quite a lot of complex partial seizures, absence seizures, simple partial seizures, and who knows how many night time seizures I might have had? No wonder people were nervous around me when it came to trying to set up my own business. I guess people have perceived me as too vulnerable to work on my own or take on that much responsibility. I did not always get warnings before a seizure which only added to my vulnerability whilst living and working in Scotland and trying to set up my own business.

I can see now why I was so depressed and home sick in Glasgow. People in Glasgow made me face up to my demons. As much as they also helped me which I appreciated; at the same time there has never been a time in my life where I felt so lonely and isolated. Now I understood why the Scottish man at my graduation told me to go home, perhaps I was enjoying myself so much in Edinburgh that I was not accepting who I was and my purpose in life. Going home meant dealing with my demons and facing who I was and to find out why I was running away. Not something I felt quite ready for but at the same time realising this was something I needed to do.

I wrote some good poetry while I was in Glasgow and I made the most of my time there knowing that at some point I would have to leave. However, I was still not sure where I was going. Since we left Manchester in 2001 mum had built a new life for herself and my friends had all moved on too. They all had their own lives, had married or had children, apart from two who still lived at home with their parents. One of these friends moved out of the area with her parents and I lost contact with her. I managed to contact her through friends reunited when I was living in Edinburgh, and found she had moved to Southport and that her mother had passed away a year after I moved to Scotland.

So moving back to Manchester in January 2003 was going to be very different for me, as there was no one there for me. If I joined my mum then I would have to move in the direction she was going in as she too had moved on. Mum had a caravan in Cumbria and she was also working in Blackpool. Since she was living with someone I would have to rent out a flat and find a job so I would be starting all over again which with more stuff than I started out with and would require a removal van. Once again I started to feel the fear and anxiety I experienced when I was a teenager but it was slightly different. This time it felt more like apprehension than the panic and phobia I had has a child. I started to learn and understand the difference which helped me understand myself in greater detail. I found I experienced my anxiety differently, although I was still anxious and nervous about going back to Manchester after three years of being away. What I found was a totally different experience. The apprehension I had experienced really was not necessary, since Manchester, Salford and even Eccles had changed. A lot had improved and I was now going back to a very different place to that which I had left behind.

For months after my course ended only having a part time job and no money meant not having much to do. Glasgow was not like Edinburgh, I needed money to venture out to the city, going for a walk or sitting in the garden was ok but now there was little left. I would meet with my friends once a week but my mind was often elsewhere. I found comfort in writing poetry and lots of inspiration in my own emotions and surroundings.

My GP made me an appointment for Glasgow General Hospital where I would see a consultant neurologist and put my epilepsy under investigation, at the same time I would undergo a series of test to see if neuro surgery was possible. Obviously I was nervous but at the same time excited as some of these tests were ones that my mum said I was meant to have done when I was a child. These were the tests that would confirm my epilepsy once and for all. After this there would be no disputing the fact and I could begin the process of accepting my condition. As medication was not something I was keen to return to, when these tests were mentioned I was so up for it. Of course if surgery was an option I would take it. Did Glasgow have any idea what it was like to live with my condition? I had so many questions.

I was unable to stay in Glasgow for the full test as by Christmas, life was getting tense at the house and all the house mates but one were gone. I knew I could not stay there any longer. My mum of course would have to move me out in two or three trips since I had managed to accumulate a lot of baggage. I would spend Christmas with mum back at the caravan before moving back to Manchester. Mum was going to look after my belongings until I got settled again. However I had no idea where I was going to stay or work since I had not thought that far ahead. May be I would just take the risk upon my return to Glasgow, for the remainder of the test, and stay at friends and have the hospital transfer me to my local hospital in Salford or Manchester depending on where ended up once I was settled. In the mean time I was going home.

Chapter Six

Back home

Back home I needed to find a job, somewhere to live and start over. Having spent Christmas with mum and her partner I spent a few extra weeks at the caravan while I got my finances in order and dealt with some paper work. However having seen the countryside I knew this was not the place I wanted to be.

So I decided to go back to the place I grew up in, check on a few friends, show my face and see what if anything had changed in the past three years. Not that three years seemed like a long time to me. However in three years there had certainly been some huge developments. For example before I moved they were building the Trafford Centre although I never did get to see them complete the project. Plus there were other developments taking place in Manchester and various other areas. So when I did come back there had been many changes. I wondered if these developments would assist me in finding work, if I could get a job then all that remained was finding somewhere to stay.

I spent the first two months staying with friends and family. I finally got a bed-sit just up the road from where I used to live which was not bad at all. It meant that I had to share my accommodation with a few others but I was used to that up in Scotland. I had been transferred back to Salford Royal Hospital and I managed to get my old job back as a part-time care assistant and a second job as a personal assistant for woman who needed some assistance in her own home. I put my name back on the housing list and settled in to life back where I grew up. I was home and it was like I had never been away.

However I soon found a repeat of the old pattern. In the first year back in my home town I went through four jobs and soon discovered that even though some members of staff or even my employers were ok with my medical condition, not everyone was as understanding. I simply either did not know how to work with the staff who were giving me a hard time or I felt that they treated me differently. I felt as though I was being bullied or discriminated against and there were simply no measurements put in place to protect me. In the end after one incident at work resulted in me giving up my job and moving out of the area; I decided that if I were to succeed in work I needed to find out my employment rights and make sure that I had some kind organisation behind me that would protect me in some way. I discovered that the charity I was once involved in was still around so I re-joined and I started attending their local epilepsy support group. I figured the more I knew about my condition and the more I knew about my rights the better chance I had of holding a job down.

The epilepsy support group would meet once a month in a pub so I would go along and get involved as much as I could. I found the group useful for a number of reasons. One guy named Ian who attended was a member of another charity that supported people who didn't work and helped with various forms and I was able to make use of the advice he gave me. Although the advice made little difference to keeping my job it proved to come in useful during the campaigns I would go on to run in the future.

I managed to get Disability Living Allowance and a bus pass sorted with Ian's help and when I finally got my own place I was armed with all kinds of information about my rights as a tenant and what kind of support I should be entitled to. However I soon found myself writing many letters to MP's after discovering that despite having rights and regulations laid out for people with disabilities, many of them are often ignored or broken or there is an overlap due to health and safety and loop holes which I found frustrating.

I hit so many brick walls while trying to fight them and often wondered whether it was due to a lack of communication or misunderstanding. Nevertheless, it left me feeling like I was being discriminated against. Is it born out of a need to protect the vulnerable that leads to such poor inequality and isolation?

Another problem I often encountered was the fact that there is simply a lack of funds available to make improvements. There have been many jobs I would have loved to have stayed in, however if it was not for the experiences I went through, I would never have made it has far as Glasgow where I got the proper diagnosis that I needed. I have always enjoyed work and the most frustrating part of this has always been the difficulty in keeping hold of a job.

During the time I was in Scotland I had also applied once more for an update of my medical records. This time however I was not approaching my GP for access to my GP's notes. I had made an application to the hospital before I moved to Scotland. Because it was the NHS and I was now campaigning and doing my own research my relationship with the

NHS had changed. I found accessing my records was not as easy as I thought it would be. I succeeded in gaining access to my records in 2000 though it took me another two years to make sense of them. I found accessing my records through the hospital was not that simple either. Although I now had a better relationship with various health professionals,(as through the various charities I was now willing to work with the hospitals to make improvements to the services), I wondered why I still came up against so many brick walls and stigmas when it came to working with various services.

As I read through my medical records I learned there was a lot of support that I received from the hospitals over the years. There was also a lot of knowledge that if it had been shared with both me and my mother, would have been of great benefit throughout my life. As none of this was ever communicated by any of the services that either me or my mother came into contact with; when I started college and began conducting my own research I found that I was asking the same questions my mother once asked. The only feeling that me and my mother ever felt was frustration. I simply spent the majority of my life going around in circles.

Having moved into my new flat I then started a new job at the local supermarket which came in handy for rent money and paying some bills. Receiving Disability Living Allowance helped too, although I did struggle as I was taking on more responsibility than I was used to. Before I was just paying towards rent and electric now I was paying for everything by myself. I had never lived completely on my own before and while I enjoyed having my own independence and space this was not only an anxious time for me but for a person with epilepsy a time of uncertainty.

I had gone from being dependent on my mother to running my own home. I guess most people see a person with epilepsy as totally vulnerable and dependant on others. I have been looked at as stupid, naive and vulnerable. People have misunderstood or misinterpreted my memory problems as confusion and many have told me that I would be incapable of achieving most things in life. I could not get away from the feeling that I had to prove myself to others due to my condition being perceived in a different light. Not everyone is reliant on others, yes we require a little help from time to time and everyone is different in terms of care needs. It is the medication that turns us into drugged up dependant people not the seizures. Yes when we have a seizure we are out of it for ten minutes at the most. Any longer than ten minutes it is time to call for an ambulance. Most people recover quickly after a seizure and are well enough to carry on with their usual duties and get on with whatever they were doing beforehand. They do not require a baby sitter. Some people I know with epilepsy are on six different types of medication and are conscious. They are coherent and capable of doing their own shopping and maintain their own homes. Others are on four different types of medications and require support to go to the shops. Everyone is different and reacts differently to the medication they receive. It all depends on each individual, so how can you treat every person that you encounter with epilepsy the same way?

I knew I needed a more secure job as the supermarket was only part time and I knew that this job would only be a temporary one until something more permanent with more cash came along; and I needed to make the most of the qualifications I had worked so hard to attain. However until then I needed to concentrate on my flat. My flat was already furnished considering the amount of stuff I had accumulated during my time in Scotland and what I already had before that. Plus my mum having done her fair share of travelling had quite a collection of furniture from at least three houses.

Therefore most of that furniture was now making its way over to mine. One day my brother just turned up with a sofa from mum's cottage down south, then mum turned up with a cooker, a kettle, a microwave and toaster. She passed on to me her old Hoover from when she was sixteen. Two deck chairs, a miniature table, an electric heater, a large TV, two rugs, a collection of pots and pans, plates and mugs, the list went on. I was sure it was my mum moving in to my flat not me, by time she finished. I think I only had to buy a bed and a few extra items to make the place my own. "We have four properties between us," Mum told me, "but we have nowhere to put all this so you can have it."

Over time most of the stuff my mother gave me went to the charity shops or I donated it to the local church or sold it. On each visit my mother said she had something more for me. I imagined her home to be like some kind of treasure trove. I kept telling my mother to have a jumble sale as I was sure she would make a profit. I had my own vision of what I wanted my place to look like and was getting fed up of my brother calling me a hoarder. I was quite happy to be involved with the various charities and campaigns. I was not happy to be seen as a charity case, hoarder or incapable of providing for myself. I already had several stigmas and assumptions to contend with though I was very appreciative of my mother for her support.

Having succeeded in getting my flat how I wanted it and getting rid of most of the clutter mum had helped me build up I managed to secure myself a decent steady job working as a post room assistant for an insurance company. I felt I was settled back in Manchester and I could start making plans again for my future.

The money was better and I thought that this job might just be the one I was looking for in terms of career prospects. With my qualifications and the work experience, I could build up my qualifications and may be work my way into teaching, running workshops or something similar to the route I wanted to follow originally. If life experience is what I was short on then I would certainly get it here. Maybe if I could hold this job down for a few years and save up I could perhaps do the courses I needed to get back on track. I definitely saw this job as a promotion. I was up front about my epilepsy and honest and open at the interview so that we could start on the right footing. The following day I got a second phone call asking me to come back for another interview followed by a training day. This was clearly good news so of course I handed in my notice to the supermarket straight away. I couldn't wait to start, the following month I was there bright and early.

I worked for the insurance company for two and half years, during which time I had a variety of experience working in different departments. I really did enjoy it, however one little detail got in the way… **my epilepsy**.

During the first year everything seemed to go well for me, even though the company were aware of my condition. I passed my six months' probation and even earned good bonuses. After the first year however, everything

73

changed. I had a seizure whilst covering reception. After which I was no longer allowed to work on reception. Then I had a few seizures in the post room. I don't ever recall the company ever carrying out a risk assessment. Yet the company started to treat me differently, everything had changed. I knew that I was no longer wanted despite no one ever saying anything out of place.

My medication changed again and I started to feel paranoid, especially in work. I felt more and more tired and my concentration started to slip. Soon I found my memory was becoming affected and I was no longer able to focus on my job. Despite this, my employer would not allow me to alter my hours, I ended up getting the Disability Discrimination Act involved and contacting my union which did not improve my relationships in work or staff morale between myself and certain work colleagues. No matter how much support various members of staff tried to give me I noticed a pattern emerging. Not everyone was playing the same game and I soon started to feel like I was being forced out. Whether or not that was just my paranoia because of the medication or fact relating to certain members of staff I don't know, but the job that I hoped would be for life soon began to fall apart. My medication not only affected my seizures at night but my ability to get up in the morning, concentrate on my work and focus during the day. As much as I tried to make my work colleagues understand I found not many businesses or organisations paid much attention or were interested in epilepsy or neurological conditions.

My night time seizures increased and I soon started to have seizures on the way to work. This increase in seizures caused me to be late, so the only way to get to work would be to get a taxi. Clearly getting taxis in to work each day was not helpful from a financial perspective, but it was the only way to make my supervisor and HR staff see that I was making an effort. I don't think they believed I was having seizures or that I missed the bus for that reason. I would even refuse the emergency service and ask the witnesses not to call the ambulance or to cancel the call so that I could go to work. The boss never believed me when I told them about the days that the bus never turned up, all they saw were the times I was clocking into work late and the days I was taking off due to hospital and doctors' appointments or due to my seizures. Clearly they were target driven and a person with uncontrollable epilepsy was not going to help them meet their targets. Eventually it was clear the job was not working out and after two and a half years (the longest I have ever held down a job) I knew I had to go. Following six months of arguments with a work colleague and a year and a half fighting my case with my employers I decided to hand in my notice.

I think I had two weeks still left to serve when an argument between me and a work colleague broke out. It was clear I'd had enough given the outcome and on this particular day itself, well, I'm not sure if it was the way I was feeling given the side effects of the medication, or the way I was feeling about work that made me do it but one minute the work colleague was raising her voice the next I had a glass of water in my hand then I recall us both standing up and the water going all over her and the computer! I do not recall the particular medication I was taking although I was aware they had weird side effects including depression, anxiety, poor concentration and paranoia. I came off that medication shortly afterwards.

Well that was the end of my career in insurance and I have no idea what they did with my work colleague but I never found paid employment afterwards. I had ago at self-employment as I felt that employers simply did not understand unseen disability. It is easier to make adaption's for a physical disability but any form of hidden disability apparently is harder to make adaption's for due to the fact that unless someone experiences the condition they have no idea what it is like. Then again, due to the large amount of closed doors it is harder to set up on your own, so how could you possibly set something up for someone else if you struggle to break through the barriers in the first place.

Being a little dyslexic, experiencing memory problems and having epilepsy would present me with many challenges. I often felt I was being treated differently in work and regardless of the many CRB checks I passed, references I obtained and interviews I sat, none of it made any difference to me because once I was in and working for whatever company took me on, I often felt everything changed once the company or organisation noticed my spelling, grammar and concentration was not up to scratch. I found I was often treated differently once people noticed my short term memory and once my seizures were noted then there was often no getting away from the obvious. I often found people I encountered in a working capacity often perceived my seizures as too much of a concern or risk; and due to health and safety legislation and the Disability Discrimination Act it was often difficult to sack me once they made the "mistake" of taking me on - regardless of the fact that I had come clean about my fainting attacks and epilepsy. I would have presented the employer with an updated copy of my CV showing all my certificates to date and references so there were no excuses when it came to my employment. However I still often felt that I was treated differently in the work place regardless of whether or not I was doing paid or unpaid work. I often felt people treated me like a liar or confused person or someone who was stupid. When it came to my dyslexia and memory problems I often found the two combined with stress and anxiety affected my spelling which in turn had a knock on effect on how others often treated me or responded. I eventually got fed up of the put downs from friends, family and work colleagues who were constantly criticising my spelling especially those who were aware of my memory problems and anxiety. In the end I began to distance myself from people I knew, even in my voluntary work and I stopped engaging with people.

Of course this did not help my self-esteem and confidence; after all I had been through when I struggled to set up a business in Scotland, improve my personal development and move forward.

So as you can see I had gone through many different jobs, and tried to set up my own business but eventually I was to discover that a combination of epilepsy and politics would obstruct the path to following my dreams. The only other option was my back up plan which was my childhood dream of writing a book.

My relationships, stigma and the criticism did not improve when I tried to get the first book published. In the end I gave up and started to approach self-publishing companies. Though they too I found were expensive; having to pay for the cost of editors, proof readers and printers. It was a self-publishing company that was to become my first experience and taste of the publishing world and it was a great learning curve for me. Although it would be an expensive process for my first book (which was not a book that would go on to sell well although I would learn a great deal from it) I had no intention of giving up on my writing career. I knew that I would probably get a few knock backs given my medical condition and dyslexia, but I had a few replies from self-publishing companies and although I was unable to afford self-publishing at that time, I found that for my poetry at least self-publishing would be the way forward for the first poetry book.

Chapter Seven

The Test Results

Back at Glasgow I spent a week under observation via a Video EEG test or telemetry test. This is basically a week of observation involving being hooked up to some wires and monitored by cameras for at least seven days. During the EEG part of the test I had electrodes stuck onto my head to monitor my brain waves and any seizure activity .The video or cameras in the room filmed any seizures that took place at the same time. I was monitored over a twenty-four hour period during which time I was not allowed to leave the room I was given. Luckily I was given my own suite so I had my own bathroom and toilet facility. I could have a shower but I was not allowed to wash my hair until the wires were removed. There was a box hooked onto a belt which was connected to an alarm system in case I had a seizure. The alarm would alert nursing staff.

The room itself was equipped with a TV, CD player (although I was advised to bring my own headphones), music, personal CD player, magazines and books to keep myself amused. Visitors were allowed in at certain times although I imagined that as I no longer lived in the Glasgow area my visitors were going to be scarce.

I only had one visitor from Glasgow during the whole time. He did come to visit twice and brought with him magazines and whatever I needed for which I was very grateful. I relied on my mobile phone for company most of the time, and I'm not sure just how long I was in there for. I did have a few seizures the day I arrived before they hooked me up to the machines and I'm not sure how many night time seizures they recorded although the nurses did catch one daytime seizure which they managed to record.

The day they "unplugged" me so to speak and I was allowed to have a shower, I was shown the video of the seizure they had recorded. To be honest, having got over the shock and slap in the face that yes you do have epilepsy and there is nothing that can be done about it, I was able to watch the video of myself with sheer amusement. There I was sitting on the hospital bed sorting out the pillows, but I was really having a go at them. I would beat them up then put them straight again, then beat them up then put them back in their place. The whole thing was actually quiet comical.

During the time I was having a seizure, the consultant and a nurse came into the room and one of them proceeded to ask me a set of questions, none of which I answered. I did not seem to acknowledge that the consultant or the nurse were present. I was talking a load of rubbish none of which made any sense yet I remained on the bed the whole time. I don't think my seizure lasted that long and after I came round the only person I was aware of was the nurse.

One thing I do have a tendency to do is to sleep afterwards. I sometimes have a headache or migraine so will sometimes sleep that off. Or, I will feel a little confused and disorientated and it can sometimes take a little longer for my memory to come back so that I can recall what it was that I was doing before the seizure occurred.

The day I was leaving hospital I was introduced to a counsellor and epilepsy specialist nurse. I had already met the team of consultants, student nurses and technicians. Now it was time to talk about my epilepsy. I had blood taken from me and had been started on some medication; and now I was expected to watch the video and talk about how I felt. Something was sounding all too familiar only this time, before I went I was going for a MRI scan and someone was going to talk to me about the possibility of surgery. I've had the tilt test done and the flashing lights test and just maybe I wouldn't mind all these trips to and from the out patients if there was the possibility of surgery.

I was informed that I was a little ambidextrous and that I have right temporal lobe epilepsy, which (after surgery) the diagnoses was changed to refractory epilepsy (resistant to medication). I was also informed that I have some scarring on the back of my brain, some fractures on the front of my skull and that my skull is too small to fit the whole of my brain in so I don't have a whole brain. Ok are they serious? I remember thinking that I'd let that one go until I saw the images for myself. Other observations included that they considered me to be slightly dyslexic, that one leg is shorter than the other and that they wondered why I have the tremors. Again I remember thinking that if they were the neurologist and the consultants why couldn't *they* tell me? Perhaps the tremors have something to do with my anxiety or constant changes to medication.

I was also informed that I had at least five different types of seizures some with warnings and some without. One or two of which I was not even aware of experiencing?

There were a lot more observations made although these were perhaps not as interesting so I think that I filed them away in the back of my mind somewhere. It was not until I was re-investigated that the test results of 2004 came back to me.

Based on the fractures to my skull and the scarring on the back of my brain, Glasgow said that neuro surgery was too risky and referred me back to Salford Royal having already started me on medication. Perhaps surgery was another possibility in the future. For now of course I had to repeat the process of trying various medications and taking regular trips to out patient's appointments to get my blood checked and see various consultants. I'm sure I had been through all this before and not much had changed.

I was however, re-diagnosed with epilepsy and assigned to a neurologist where I would attend for regular appointments. I found the investigation and experience reassuring and felt at peace and was happy with the team of consultants that had looked after me. Unfortunately though, surgery was not an option for me and I was now back on medication. I agreed to give medication another go for a few more years although I was not looking forward to the side effects. At the same time I did not like the seizures and the experiences I'd had which had affected my career. I wanted my condition stabilised and had reached a point where I was willing to give anything a go to gain back some control of my life.

At least I would be given a proper diagnosis and would get to see what my seizures looked like and maybe I would get to try again in a few years' time perhaps through a different hospital. In the mean time I concentrated on my own research and found out what I could on the internet. I was hoping there would be something either myself or the doctors had missed or may be having my own knowledge would help me when I next paid a visit to my consultant?

It was through this research that I found a forum where people with epilepsy could meet up via the Epilepsy Action website. So I joined it in the hope that there was a network of people and more knowledge I could learn from them. However, I found myself sitting reading through the website's information and just reading posts asking the same questions that at first were bothering me.

Each time I went to post on the forum it seemed that the post had already been posted by someone else, and I found dozens of posts written many times by many people all asking the same questions :-

"Clearly these are the answers the consultants should be giving and may be even the kind of information the consultants themselves ought to have access to."

82

So rather than asking the same questions I started taking notes with the intention of putting these questions to the consultants on my next visit.

What I found interesting was that when I went to the doctors and consultants armed with my information the relationship between me and the consultants seemed to change. I ended up having many arguments with some of my specialists. I would often make use of the internet, write letters to various organisations and charities and do a wide range of research in order to back up my theories. Although it helped me to understand myself and my own condition I found it was not always helpful during my consultations to take my research with me. It turned out that they were no more the wiser than me, most were just learning and as we the patients learned more about our condition so did the consultants. They were no different than us and I found I was now on a whole new learning curve only this time with the hospital.

This took me on a new adventure! I started doing research not just for the hospitals but for the charities. I started getting involved with campaigns through a range of charities and organisations most of which was done online. I did not mind sharing as I got to know more people through networking. I started attending conferences, campaigns and taking my campaigns further into my writing. I found my relationship changed again with the NHS and hospital. I was no longer feeling frustrated at not getting anywhere as I now felt I was on the same learning curve as the hospital and the rest of the staff. I no longer felt the need to attend the GP and regular out patient's appointments unless I had new information I felt would help the hospital with their own research. I began buying books off the internet and from bookshops and spending time researching. Sometimes I would get frustrated that my research did not get me any further, then at other times I would feel a sense of achievement although this was rare.

Later on, the research I was involved in would be beneficial to the hospital and other hospitals throughout the UK. In the future they would welcome my research and research from others although it would take some time before the hospital would see the benefits.

Chapter Eight

London

In 2009 I was back on benefits with no job and my own flat, not a position I wanted to be in. When I moved back to Manchester the intention was to set up again and may be put my qualifications to good use. Instead my seizures were out of control. I had one seizure by the kitchen window; bearing in mind I lived ten floors up and anything could have happened to me. I came round on the bathroom floor once or twice and woke up one morning with bruises on my arms. I had no idea where the bruises came from. I had been diagnosed with depression and I felt like chucking myself out of the kitchen window next time I came to stand by it.

I was struggling with my depression and although I knew that a combination of antidepressants and antiepileptic medication was unlikely to work, I tried it anyway. Although I tried to fight my case it was no use, the job centre encouraged me to apply for income support. I knew about the tribunal service but had no idea how to go about it, so I found myself taking the job centre's advice. As a result I found myself taking more of an interest in the campaign work through the various charities I was now involved in. I did not have an understanding of politics at this time but coming out of work for a final time marked the start of my campaign work and my journey into self-employment.

It was back to the doctors again for a review and another appointment with the neuro, as clearly the medication was not working, and something had to be done.

Back at the hospital after a long discussion with the consultant I was offered a choice of a Vagus Nervous Stimulator (VNS) being fitted at Salford Royal or being referred to a professor at one of London's hospitals to have another bash at neuro surgery. I turned down the offer of VNS I had a few friends who had them inserted and had read about others on various internet sites and I didn't fancy a battery been placed inside me and all the messing about that it involved especially if it got turned off for some reason or I had to go through the whole thing again five or ten years down the line.

At least with neuro surgery even though it was a risky operation I had heard so many positive things about it and this was something I had always wanted. If I went to London then at least I would get a definite "yes"or "no" answer to confirm if surgery was an option for me. If I was not a suitable candidate I could look at the VNS at a later date.

To have the operation was a once in a life time opportunity for me that could give me the freedom to be seizure free. Despite what Glasgow told me back **in 2003** I believed that the brain can change along with a person's epilepsy. Technology had advanced and London had the best. An appointment was made for me in February to go to London and meet the consultant who would be taking care of me from now on and after that appointment a further appointment was made for me to attend the National Society for Epilepsy down in Chalfont, Buckinghamshire to start the test.

I was hopefully on the way to big changes, it was another new adventure. I was filled with lots of excitement and anxiety at the same time as I had never been to a hospital purely dedicated to people with epilepsy. I was not sure what to expect. The research, documentaries and books I had read had prepared me and I was armed with lots of useful information and knowledge ready for the doctors. I already knew that I had drug resistant epilepsy where my condition simply does not respond to medication, and I was too sensitive to a lot of medication available. Despite this people would often suggest that I try something else and to go back on medication and be on medication the rest of my life. Neuro surgery for me was the last option. I already knew through films and documentaries I seen over the years that not everyone responded to this form of treatment. I had met people who had neuro surgery and I knew there were a small minority who had surgery and it had worked. I knew the risk but what I wanted more than ever was to be seizure free.

Mum came with me and she was also excited as she too felt that I was finally getting my health looked into and sorted out; finally someone was listening to her and paying some attention. We took the train into London as London is a very big city and we had no idea how far the hospital we were attending would be. However, we found the hospital very easily and only had a twenty minute walk from Euston Station. The hospital itself was a huge university hospital split into various sections and I didn't realise just how chaotic the place would be.

Even though we were half an hour early for our appointment we seemed to be waiting for ages. When we did finally go into see the professor I had been referred to, I found the experience to be nothing like I imagined. I found this particular professor to be quite down to earth and laid back, although he clearly knew his job well and was quite straight forward about it. He certainly did not hide any detail when discussing any fears or concerns. I knew then our relationship might be a little bumpy at times but that he was the consultant I wanted to work with. I found the professor to be knowledgeable, caring and on my level. Out of all the consultants and doctors I had met over the years I actually felt comfortable and at home with this one and I knew we would get along well. Later on I would meet the professor again at Chalfont during the first phase of testing.

At the National Society for Epilepsy (**NSE**) it was like driving into a city or town in its own right. On site there was a B&B, community centre, residential flats, day care facility, out-patients hospital, GP surgery, restaurants, hospice, residential home, and various other facilities as the grounds were designed for people who were visiting on a day to day basis. **The NSE** is the national society for epilepsy a charity based organisation and works with the London based hospitals to offer care and support for people with epilepsy.

I was staying in an area called Chalfont and mum was staying on site in the B&B for the few days that I was there. I shared a room with two other girls, one of which I was to become good friends with. She would be someone I would remain in contact with throughout my journey through neuro surgery. The unit I was staying in had various communal areas and places where other patients could socialise or places where we could be alone. I found that I came to enjoy my time in Chalfont; although at times some of my future visits, even the shorter ones would be visits I couldn't wait to get away from no matter how short my stay was. This one was the main essential stay and I didn't mind even though my last appointment was with the psychologist and I spent most of my time on the bed in tears. This was mainly due to the realisation that I discovered why my memory was as bad as it was and some aspects of the test that I should have found easy I simply could not do. I see now why my job with the insurance company did not work out. Perhaps if I had received a diagnosis of my memory back then they would have had a better understanding, or maybe they simply would never have employed me as they would have known from looking at my results that there is no way I could have met those targets.

Perhaps from the test results the hospital would know how my memory would work after surgery. No wonder people thought they could take advantage! I still remember how many times my friends would ask if I could lend them money and then not give it back; or how often my friends thought they could take advantage by asking me to pay for something and they would give me the money later. Or that they would post me the difference as they didn't have the money at that moment. It's not just that part of my short term memory is damaged, some of my long term memory has been affected; but just because I have epilepsy doesn't mean I am thick and stupid. So for any of you "friends" who are reading this book, you know who you are, I have not forgotten and someday karma will catch up with you even if I don't.

As for other tests, having had my psychology, MRI and blood test I had an appointment with psychiatry and that was followed up by the consultant and specialist nurse before I spent time with the professor who talked about the next appointment. I was put on the waiting list for a second video telemetry test only this time I was having it done in London. Unlike the one I had done in Glasgow I would stay on a ward with others and we would share the bathroom and a toilet facility, the only thing dividing us was a curtain. My consultant would write to Glasgow for my previous video EEG results and have a look at them. In the mean time I would go down to London when called and prepare myself for a second test.

When I the appointment date it came through it was the beginning of summer in **June**, I remember the day well. I was packing for London when I had the terrible feeling something was wrong. In my gut there was a terrible tragedy occurring elsewhere in the world, although I felt that I didn't want to know about it. I had experienced a premonition dream a week earlier and I had a feeling it was something to do with my idol **Michael Jackson**. Michael had announced various tour dates in March earlier that year and I knew then that it was not going to happen.

I tried to get tickets and when I couldn't get tickets I knew it simply was not meant to be. In my heart I had already said good bye. I turned up my music and continued packing. I tried ignoring the fact that the house phone was playing up all afternoon. I had already worked my way through my phone list to see if anyone had been trying to phone me. BT could not work out a fault on my phone and I couldn't figure out why the TV stations were playing up. By 11pm I couldn't take anymore and I turned on the television to watch a film on True Movies. I felt that someone was trying to tell me something. Eventually, at midnight text messages started coming through. In my premonition dream a week earlier I had seen Michael Jackson's bedroom and his bed, I had seen the train journey I was going to take and the news reports, everything that morning happened the way I had seen it, starting with the text messages and the phone call to one of my friends who was the first person to text me.

After I heard confirmation from one of my friends that my premonition had come true I had no choice but to switch on the news and contact my mum. I was awake all night. Not a good thing depriving myself of sleep when I was about to travel to London for a video EEG. Or was it? There was talk of some sleep deprivation during that week to try and bring on a seizure. So maybe I got the ball rolling there? Not that I wanted a seizure on the train to London just in case I did not make it to the right hospital or ward on time.

On the train to London that morning of course every newspaper on every front page confirmed the news that my idol had passed away. I'm not sure if I was in shock or simply stunned. It was news I had expected and I always knew my idol would never live to be an old man, despite the fact that he was someone I looked up to and had been a fan of ever since I was the age of eight or ten.

Once in London I found that the hospital was within walking distance of the rail station; and the ward I was booked to spend the next week on was not that bad either. Although I had to share a ward we each had dividers separating us in order to provide a degree of privacy, although it was nothing like the room I had up in Glasgow. I was going to be in the end cubicle. My friend from London would be down at some point to visit me once I was settled in and she would phone or text me on a regular basis. I found the staff were very friendly and I had a good view over London from the window at my bedside. Not that I would be paying much attention to the view of London, my friend brought me some newspapers and magazines to read though I spent most of the week glued to the news and taking in the message of Michael Jackson's death. A UFO could have landed that week and I would not have noticed. If I was not listening to the news then I was playing my videos, DVD's or listening to Michael's music. It wasn't until the week was over that I met the guy in the next cubicle and a comment was made on my music and DVD's.

That poor patient and the hospital staff must have felt like they were at a concert not in a hospital. Of course I had my head phones with me and at times I did use them although it was obvious who the Michael Jackson fan was on the ward! As for the video EEG test the staff did not record any day time seizures this time though they did record a few night time and sleep seizures. I had more seizures after leaving the hospital, I think I found the hospital environment relaxing, despite being in shock and having little sleep the night before I arrived. It was clear from the EEG that I have more night time seizures than I have in the day; although I am not always aware of the night time or sleep seizures unless I wake up having just come out of one, or feeling groggy or tired after waking up. Sometimes I might feel like I have a hangover first thing in the morning although I don't drink a lot of alcohol. If I wake up feeling like I have a hangover and I know I have not been drinking the night before then I know it must have been a result of a seizure. Other than feeling extra tired and needing more sleep, I do not have any other evidence for night time seizures unless I wake up with blood on my pillow or bedding and I know the blood has not come from my mouth. Or I wake up with scratch marks on parts of my body, or bruises with no other explanation other than a seizure in the night where I grabbed myself or hurt myself on something.

If a person with epilepsy lives on their own then it is very difficult to collect evidence of seizures unless there is physical evidence such as bruises or injuries that need medical attention or that person can remember going into or coming out of the seizure. It's only then that we can keep a seizure diary and record them for the hospital. Apart from that we rely on others for evidence. This is why we need more people to understand more about epilepsy especially when you consider the dangers.

After my video telemetry test at the hospital in London I had a second appointment with my consultant at the University College London Hospital (UCLH) to go through the test results. This was followed by a further MRI scan and other tests at the NSE in Chalfont. Here the tests got more intense especially when the psychology test gave me the first impression of what my mind was like.

The MRI scan might have shown me what my brain looked like, which I found interesting; but I was more concerned with understanding why it was like it is and how my mind worked. That helped me understand my epilepsy in more detail. I found out more about my condition this way. I had been diagnosed with right temporal lobe epilepsy, now I wanted to know what that meant and the psychology test put a lot into perspective for me though I did get frustrated at the test and I found a lot of what we did in that room hard going.

A person with right temporal lobe epilepsy has difficulty with spacial awareness and their brain works differently and absorbs information in a different way to a person whose mind or brain is not damaged. **(See Barry J Gibb, "The Rough Guide to the Brain" Rough Guides Reference Titles 2007).** Temporal lobe epilepsy is associated with sound, vision, language, emotion, and visual-spatial processing. So did this explain why I've always been an emotional person, had difficulty with directions, using maps, had problems with my memory and absorbing information regardless of the medication and seizures? Or is the amount of medication I've been on over the years and the seizures to blame?

My brain had not developed properly prior to my birth, and when I was born there was also an element of stress which might have contributed to this theory. I also discovered that as each seizure slowly ate away at my cells my brain had to find new pathways which meant new memories and learning processes. I have always struggled with memory problems and as I have grown older my memory has worsened. The noticeable one was my short term memory and concentration. Although a combination of stress, anxiety and seizures was to blame, temporal lobe damage was not the only brain damage I encountered. I found out through tests I also had right optical lobe damage which would explain the problems with my vision and focus. Effects of my seizures were also evident on my hippocampus which may cause other problems if the surgeons were to operate.

I've always been a spiritual person and have always been very intuitive, experiencing premonitions and visions about the future. I am probably being shown something that is going to happen or link me to someone or an event that will happen ten years down the line. Sometimes I just "knew" something would happen or experience coincidences. There were many events that took place over the years that I did not understand until later on. **Gibb's** book however, would argue that my epilepsy and the fact that my right brain is the side with the most seizure activity is responsible for the "visual hallucinations." Or, as the neurologist would call them "visual distortions." I have to dispute this as epilepsy may run in my dad's side of the family, but not in my mother's side and I know that there are a lot of

94

people on my mother's side who are very intuitive and gifted, also experiencing telepathy and premonitions. I know a lot of people who do not have epilepsy and are what I would call gifted. So I try not to say too much about my spiritual side to the doctors, consultants or psychologists when I'm at the hospital, which is hard as the "gifts" as I call them are part of me.

Once I had had the entire safe test I was sent back home to await an invitation to go back to London to meet with the neuro surgeon. In the mean time I had a lot of thinking to do. I now knew what my brain looked like, I had a proper diagnosis and I knew that neuro surgery may be an option for me. In the mean time I had an appointment with my specialist nurse in Manchester and a referral for cognitive behaviour therapy at a community centre nearby to help me with my decision for neuro surgery.

I had seen all the specialists while in London. Now I wanted to check with myself that I was making the right decision and try to gain my family's support. The rest of the year was going to be tough.

In the mean time I would throw myself into as much charity work as possible and socialise with as many friends as I could. If I was going to go down the surgery route the following year then I would make the most **of 2009**. I wrote a will and filled in a brain donation form. I wanted to leave my books to charity and have the hospital make the most out of me if I was not successful in recovering from the surgery. I was never afraid of death given that I had a lot of experience with death whilst working in a caring and nursing capacity. Sometimes death got me down but I did not mind since my beliefs were spiritual and I believe that the spirit lives on after death. I felt that I would survive the surgical investigation though I was unable to see beyond this. I also suffered from depression and from time to time I often felt so down, that I did think about death and contemplated suicide. There was one occasion I stood by my kitchen window thinking about my cousin who took his own life. I forget now just how long I was standing outside the kitchen window. Something made me close the kitchen window; it was the thought of surviving death that made me change my mind. I had survived so many dangerous situations with my seizures I knew I would survive neuro surgery. I was meant to be on earth for a reason, so I would go through with the investigations in order to get some answers. I really hoped that neuro surgery would be an option for me and I really did hope there was a cure.

Chapter Nine

A New Adventure

June 2010 was a weird month for me, it was the month I was seeing the neuro surgeon on my own; and I was also meeting up with my friend from London again. I had not seen her since **June 2009** when we first met in Chalfont. It seemed strange how it was all around the same time that my idol Michael Jackson passed away. A lot had happened to both of us since and we had a lot to catch up on. We were both so busy we didn't have that much time to chat.

I was also going back to Chalfont for some more tests so I felt all over the place that week, mainly due to the fact I was bad with my seizures the week before which was adding to all the stress and pressure around my week in London.

Towards the end of the week in London it was also the first anniversary of Michael Jackson's death and fans from the internet had arranged a gathering outside the O2 Arena. So I also wanted to go to that before I went home. Part of me felt like I was experiencing Deja-Vu of the year before, the only difference being that I would not be spending the whole week in a video telemetry ward. I would be visiting three hospitals in the space of two weeks and meeting hundreds of people in three different parts of England.

The month started with a huge cluster of seizures preventing me from going out the week before I was due to go to London, but my anxiety changed and I knew I had to get out and about. At some point I needed to go shopping because I had been away and not got round to doing my shopping since I returned. Given the fact I was off to London soon I thought it wise just to do a week's shopping and not buy too much. However I only made it have far as the post office to fill in a form and I suddenly found myself on the floor surrounded by two strangers. Since I had knocked myself out through hitting my head on a notice board on the wall I felt it best to go to the hospital.

Not that I was aware of any injuries at the time. Some part of me consented to an ambulance being called as I had apparently asked for one not that I remember. Sometimes during a seizure or whilst recovering or coming round from a seizure I might suffer from some memory loss though this is only temporary. I can also appear to be conscious and talking though I am not aware of what I am saying or of my surroundings and although conscious I am extremely vulnerable. I may seem like I am alert and coherent even though I am not. It is always best to check my awareness and alertness before taking anything I say during a seizure as truth or as gospel. I could be agreeing to anything which scares me knowing how this can be abused.

The next day my brother came for me and dropped me of at my flat, I was aware of my head feeling sensitive and it turned out to be a little bruised though there were no obvious injuries. My mum spent the weekend with me and I seemed to recover by the Tuesday when I was capable of getting the train down to London and make my way to my friend's house. Apparently during that weekend I had endured quite a few seizures and some pretty bad ones which made me think that either my seizures were now getting worse or had taken a different form.

Once I was at my friend's house in London, we discussed our seizures and tried to make head or tail of them. However, neither of us could figure out any answers, nor make any sense of them. If we couldn't then we guessed that the consultants, neuro surgeons and scientists were no closer.

Wednesday morning was my second interaction with a hospital only this time it was for my appointment with the neuro surgeon. My friend from London came with me as her appointment with the consultant was an hour later. It never dawned on me to ask her to come and sit in with me. So there I was alone with a new stranger, who would be responsible for removing the top of my scalp and attaching neurons, or probes which would hopefully tell him where the seizure activity was coming from. If I gave my consent.

Well this guy seemed ok, but should I trust him to open up my skull and cut my head open to place probes, then sew me back up and leave me like that for a round three weeks? Do I put my life in his hands or is this the point where I say "enough is enough I like my head the way it is thank you"?I had to take into account the last few weeks and how the epilepsy was now starting to affect me. Plus I had just knocked myself out on the wall of the post office and I had no memory of it. In addition while in my mum's car I had another seizure and I've been known to open car doors whilst having seizures in cars!

I also had a seizure while my mum stayed over and I don't remember that one.
So if I don't remember going into these seizures I just come round in a confused state and wonder who these people are and what is going on, then am I safe? The seizures were now becoming as dangerous as the operation I was contemplating.

The neuro surgeon was kind enough to show me the map of my brain on his computer once again and talk me through the process, so everything seemed straight forward.

This was not the actual split brain operation its self but an investigation to see if surgery was possible, if the probes the neuro surgeon put in found a

99

focal point then the neuro surgeon would discuss with me once again the possibility of operating in that area. So this was like the pre op to see if the actual operation was possible. Trying to explain this to my mum was not going to be easy although I would try.

After waiting for my friend we went for lunch then sat in the garden outside the hospital for a while until it was time for my friend to go to her next appointment and for me to catch the train to Chalfont for the remainder of my test. I would stay in Chalfont for a few days before getting the train to the O2 in London to be with the rest of the Michael Jackson fans for the **"MJ Vigil"** as we called it. So I did not have time to digest everything until I got home; I guess that is when I had time to think over my hospital visits and what was said.

Making the decision to have the intracranial surgery was an easy one, telling my mum was the difficult bit.

Chapter Ten

Making New Friends

Now that the tests were over and the main part of the hospital investigations were complete I could concentrate on promoting my book and trying to sell it. I also wanted to focus on meeting up with people who understood my condition or understood me; or at least start networking with people who shared the same interest. I was finding with all the stress I was under and the changes in seizures, I was moving in a different direction from my school and college friends; and even friends that I grew up with or knew from my teenage years.

In 2009 I had joined Facebook with the intention of networking and raising awareness about epilepsy. Quite a few people from the epilepsy forum joined me there too, where I got to know their real names and see their faces. At this point I still had not met any of them physically, the only contact we had was the internet. The odd one lived locally and got involved with our support group or came to the conferences. If the person on the forum worked for Epilepsy Action then I would occasionally email them or chat to them on the phone or read about them if they sent in stories to the magazine. This allowed me to take my awareness campaign and research I been doing since the age of fifteen one step further.

However, an opportunity to meet up with people from the website came shortly after I returned from London. I still had things on my mind and I needed a night out in Manchester. The forum had arranged a group get together in Manchester and around thirty people from the website came along for the weekend. This gave me a chance to discuss my concerns, fears and anxieties about surgery, the probes test and even how I felt about family not understanding. I was able to meet up with people who had recently had neuro surgery and those who had neuro surgery several years ago. They presented a variety of experiences to listen to. Putting faces to names and meeting up with people from Facebook and the forum was a great experience which I really enjoyed.

I even found myself being calm and noticing the first signs of a seizure when a person was going into one, the fact that I was in a room full of people with epilepsy did not bother me in the slightest; in fact I felt at ease. I found that these people were full of knowledge, experience and all from different walks of life. The funny thing I noticed was that the image I built up for most people was completely incorrect. I learned not to judge and just to be myself and go with the flow of life. The group from the web forum met in Manchester on the first weekend in July and I spent most of the weekend with various members of the forum chatting and going shopping. On the Friday and Saturday night we went for a meal and I spent a great deal of time getting to know the people I had spent most of my time chatting to on the internet and familiarising myself with their faces.

This interaction with other likeminded people proved really helpful, especially when I had to make the decision as to whether or not to go forward with the Intracranial Electrode Recording test; which was essential in order to locate the focal point in my brain where my seizure activity was coming from.

After the weekend I received a letter from the neuro surgeon in London that I had visited recently to discuss the surgery and the latest test. The letter dated 23rd June explained everything we had discussed at the last appointment and requested that I give my written consent to go ahead with the final test. I now needed to think about what it was that I wanted to do and if neuro surgery was what I really wanted, given that the risks associated with this test were similar to neuro surgery. Also there were some complications as my right hemisphere was covered in a white mass due to damage from birth and seizure activity. In addition, seizures were now also occurring on the back of my brain which was responsible for vision and memory. So I had a lot to talk to my new found friends about and a lot to consider.

I decided to go down to Cheltenham to visit a friend I made on a social networking site who had been through the operation I had been considering back in 2002.The meeting with her was important to me, as I knew that she now had tunnel vision and weakness down the left side of her body following a stroke that she suffered shortly after her surgery. Although she had her surgery on the left temporal lobe I felt that visiting her would help my decision and would also help my mum understand why the surgery was so important to me, when it came to discussing this with her. My mum still felt that surgery was only going to make me worse and take away my independence. Although my brother had started to come round to the idea I still felt there was a great distance to go in convincing my mother.

My mum and I have always been close, although now she was living down south and I only ever really got to see her if I was going to London for an appointment. I felt we were becoming more and more distant and the prospect of my neuro surgery was not helping matters.

In the meantime I had another drop down seizure. This seizure resulted in another visit to A&E and this time the hospital would not let me out. My brother had to come and collect me, and drop me off at home the next day. So I decided that I would probably write my letter of consent and arranged a visit to meet up with Lucy in Cheltenham. I guess the seizure was a wake-up call to the dangers my seizures were now presenting and I also realised that my seizures were changing and getting worse. Many people I spoke to who had gone ahead with neuro surgery were fine and even those who still experienced seizures after their operation had a better life than they had before surgery. Even those who experienced problems with their sight found ways of dealing with their lack of sight, or poor sight.

August was a busy month for me I had a book to promote as well as try to sell.

As well as arranging to go down to Cheltenham Spa, at the same time I would use August to catch up with my friends in Scotland who I had not seen for a few years. As well as this I had arranged with a few people on Facebook to go down to London for what would have been Michael Jackson's 52nd birthday.

My book was also complete though there were some errors that I was not happy about. However I could not afford to pay for any more corrections to be made and therefore had no choice but to settle with the minor errors and hope that people would not be too critical and see beyond this. As I had learned the hard way about self-publishing I was eager to get my book out before the operation and publish my poetry. I would use my time in Scotland to do this plus send of a few copies to friends and family in the hope that I would get some good reviews in exchange. I was also hoping that some of the epilepsy charities would offer to sell my book on their websites, and that I could help to support these charities in that way.

Meeting the girl in Cheltenham Spa turned out to be positive. She had been through a similar operation to the one I was looking into, so I was interested to see how neurosurgery had affected her and how she coped. I learned a lot from our meeting plus I got to see just how independent she was. If I had not known that she had epilepsy then I would never have guessed from meeting with her that she had. Of course there were a few little details that gave an indication of some of the side effects of neuro surgery, although one could argue that epilepsy medication could be responsible. I noticed she had a few memory problems; we could have the same conversation over again at times although I knew that medication and seizures could cause this regardless of whether or not a piece of brain had been removed.

As I had experienced memory problems and got confused at times and I understood that anyone without a medical condition can experience memory problems as part of the ageing process, this did not worry or concern me. I also met the girl's mum who had a different take on things. However, it should be taken into account that a mother or any family member would go through a lot just caring for a person with epilepsy; so I listened to what her mum had to say although I did not look too deeply into it. Just like when I met my friend from London and her mum, I found I was able to make my own conclusions as I found two great friends here who had both gone through so much. If only people could see epilepsy from our perspective as well. I guess parents get just as frustrated as we do and they think they're doing the best for us at the time, as much as we love them and can see their point of view, sometimes we need to give them a break.

So with the potential risk of haemorrhage, infection, paralysis down the left hand side of my body, my vision in the left side in both eyes, I agreed to three weeks in hospital with wires in my head, having to shave off half my locks and looking like an alien. A second operation would also be required to remove the probes. I was however, willing to take the risk since I lived with epilepsy every day and the risk of dying from a seizure whilst asleep (SUDEP) or the risk dying from my injuries. I had already experienced three head injuries this year, and I have no idea how many head injuries I have had in my life time. I figured that if I knew five people who have had neuro surgery already and two who have had the probes test then perhaps neuro surgery was not something to fear.

Lucy like Tina is someone I am proud of, as I know what both girls have gone through. Meeting people like this makes me surprised that epilepsy does not get more support; and that the neuro surgeons and hospitals offering this kind of treatment, support and care for those who have neurological conditions do not get more recognition or sponsorship. I do get very angry when I find people still struggling to get what they want in life and being treated like dirt on someone's shoe by a variety of organisations - not just people who do not understand epilepsy but by people who just do not want to help or support or are ignorant to the cause.

I wanted to be seizure free to enable me to have a normal life and be able to do everything I always dreamed of doing. I was not satisfied with my first poetry book, so I set about working on improving it and selling the book to recover my costs. I found that even in the world of publishing I was not able to get where I wanted to be and I did not always have the money to do what I wanted.

I found waiting around for an operation not just exciting but nerve wracking. I got a lot of support from a friend who had been through the process already and had a much more complicated case than mine. Although I had seen a friend go through brain surgery and be successful with his operation, making my own decision was not that easy. Just writing the consent letter was hard enough. As much as I wanted the operation and as if the stress I had already put myself through was not already enough I still had to write a consent letter. I had dreams and ambitions and wanted to do so much more with my life yet I knew that there were so many risks involved with a surgical investigation such as having my brain exposed to put electrodes on my head just so that the doctors could be sure they were operating in the right place and they might not even perform the actual operation there and then. I might find myself going through the process just to be told I couldn't have an operation or have to go through the process again. There was so much going through my mind that writing a consent letter was the hardest part of the three year investigation.

Chapter Eleven

The Consent Form

I understood that the focus of my epilepsy was on my hippocampus and that in order to get to it, the neurosurgeon would have to remove that part of my brain and disconnect my right occipital lobe. In addition, because I have right temporal lobe epilepsy and because there were two other points in my right brain where the seizures were spreading to, the surgeons would want to remove part of my right temporal lobe. This would be a six hour operation with a lot of risk attached to it.

When I first embarked on this journey back **in 2009** I wanted to go down the neuro surgery route. I knew that if there was the slightest chance I could have neuro surgery I would take it regardless of the risk. I had been living with epilepsy all my life and it brought me nothing but unhappiness. **The first video EEG** I had in Glasgow **back in 2002/ 2003** confirmed my epilepsy and I had many **MRI scans** and **EEGS**. **The second video EEG** I had in London was more detailed and the test in Chalfont showed how **poor my memory was** and what damage there was to my brain.

I now also understood that I was born prematurely and that my brain had not formed fully as my skull was too small which may have caused the scarring and the seizures. This could also have been the main stress trigger that I have had to learn to manage over the years.

Also the detailed intracranial EEG had confirmed that **I was partially blind** in one eye, which opticians don't always pick up on, probably from birth, although I rarely notice this as it is something I am now used to. I now also knew that the **seizures** had killed off the right hemisphere as the right half of my brain was nothing but a white mass; and that in the back of my brain the occipital lobe - apart from protecting my vision - had no function as it was squashed. I felt so much better– not! Learning that my seizures were now working their way across to the left side of my brain killing off brain cells as they worked their way along…

I already had two friends in hospital or supported accommodation as their epilepsy had taken their memory and they no longer knew who they were. I had two friends who had passed away; one a result of a seizure and the other I am not sure if it was sudden death due to her epilepsy, or sleep apnoea as she had both. However with such knowledge making the decision to go ahead with this operation was a difficult one although you can no doubt see why I was so angry and upset.

Over time I have learned to overcome this anger and live with and accept my condition. Though I still found there was the stigma to contend with as there were still those that believed that if you had a condition like epilepsy or some kind of brain damage then you must have either a learning condition or mental health condition. I have never believed in the tick box system as I have never fitted either category and I know a lot of other people who have similar neurological and brain conditions or conditions triggered by stress who do not fit into either category. Not everyone fits into these box systems and not everyone with a medical condition has either a learning condition or mental illness or mental health condition. I passed the point of anger and decided I would play the game for a while until I found some other way around teaching people the difference. What frustrated me was that there was little support for those who did not fit into any of these two tick box systems.

On 16ᵗʰ November 2010 I received a letter explaining what would happen once I went into hospital for the intracranial EEG. I carried the letter around with me for three days once I received it. When I eventually read the letter, I sat and cried.I was not sure if they were tears of relief that the letter had arrived, bereavement over the loss of a condition I been living with all my life or swapping my epilepsy for being visually impaired. The contents of the letter were hard to swallow. 30% chance of stopping my seizures, 15% chance of reducing or slowing my seizures down or a 5% chance that my seizures could get worse. In addition I would be guaranteed to lose my vision in the left side in both eyes and would see nothing to the left. Reading this statement alone although I already knew this would happen is what brought about the tears. That was before I turned over the page. So, could I consent to this operation? Did I really want to go ahead knowing all of this and the fact that this operation would drastically change my life?

I was up all night trying to write my consent letter. I did however manage to write a letter with pen and paper but I spent pages rambling on before I finally went to sleep. When I phoned my friend up the next day and read the letter out we both laughed at the letter's content. Later that weekend I phoned my brother who suggested I email my neuro surgeon though even this proved a difficult task. Clearly I was not ready to consent to such a risky operation and needed more time to think over what I wanted to do…

After a few days of thinking about this and anxious dreams I found the strength and courage to type up my consent letter and seal the envelope, all

I needed to do now was to send it off. Anything from here on was unknown, although in my heart I still felt positive about what I was doing and still had a good feeling about my future.

So I increased my medication and started the antidepressants and had a few appointments with various psychiatrists and other therapists. Mum obviously was waiting for me to pull out of the surgery. Either that or she thought I was going to have a long wait. I got a bit confused at one stage because even when I told mum I had given my written consent and was now on the waiting list for the first phase of neuro surgery, I was unsure if mum had actually taken it all in. I found talking about this to mum really difficult as the date of the surgery drew closer.

In June 2010, having made the decision to go through with the intracranial EEG and given my consent; I was now going to see an actual neuro surgeon to go over everything once again that I had gone through with the professor. Only this time I would be under the care of the neuro surgeon. From now on I would go to the meetings either with my friend Tina or on my own.

In April I was placed on the waiting list for the surgery. It was now just a matter of time before I was called upon to go into hospital. At the same time I would see a neuro psychologist a neuro psychiatrist and undertake therapy sessions to ensure that I was mentally and emotionally prepared for the surgery I was awaiting.

Each letter or phone call that was expected I waited for anxiously. I was the same when my appointments were due. I would leave my home two or three hours early and get the earliest or first train out. If possible I would arrange to stay over at my friend's house in London or at a guest house in London the day before my appointment.

I did as much research as possible about my forthcoming surgery and gathered as much information as I could which would help me understand the process or enable me to ask the neuro surgeon or the professor questions. I bought books, contacted the British Medical Association and even Google the medical terminology that the hospital staff and consultants used. I found myself questioning staff on a level that was sometimes beyond the doctors' expectations. If there was some other way of treating my condition without the intervention of medication or causing too much damage during surgery then I wanted and needed to know. Though prevention is often better than cure.

I did not mind engaging in medical research either or even allowing the hospital to share any medical care or research that took place while I was in their care, if it could help someone else with epilepsy in the future or assist my own care.

Tests involved in preparation for the intracranial EEG were:

- FMRI scan
- Video EEG
- Psychology
- Medical

Chapter Twelve

Neuro Surgery

I received a phone call in December, a few weeks before Christmas and was given the date of 9th January 2011 to go into hospital. However though I was both nervous and excited I was also ill with a cold. It meant staying indoors throughout Christmas and I was unable to go down to my Mums to celebrate her 50th birthday. I was advised to stay indoors and if there was no improvement to my health, then I risked cancelling the operation I been waiting for all my life. I began to wonder at this stage if there was someone out there trying to tell me something. I had written my letter of consent back in October and had many sessions with a local psychotherapist to help me make my decision. I knew I had many years left in me and that having the intracranial investigation would help to give me answers to many of the questions I have been asking over the years. Christmas was miserable but I got better, and on 9th January 2011, mum took me to London where I was checked into a ward and prepared for surgery the following day.

On the day of my arrival in hospital I was introduced to a technician who shaved off clumps of my hair and mapped out where the surgeons were going to be operating.

Before I made it to the hospital I managed to get myself to the hair dressers in January to get my hair cut. I wanted to get my hair cut short so that the neuro surgeons did not make much of a mess. My thinking was that I could still have some kind of "style". How naive was I even though I had seen some of my friends end up resulting to cutting their hair short or even shaving it all off after surgery? I thought if I cut my hair into a short bob even shaving it at the back I would still have some kind of trendy hair style after surgery. I am certain that surgeons must have some kind of banter when cutting patients' hair. The hospital would make a fortune if only they had a salon inside the hospital for patients to use on departure.

We explained to my mum the process of what would happen and where I would be sent once I had undergone surgery. We told her how long the operation would take and how long I would be in hospital for. I don't think mum could quite take it all in.

I know I put mum through three weeks of hell. I don't think even at this stage it had sunk in for my mum. I remember my mum unpacking my bags and me telling her I was not even sure I would be staying on the ward.

On 10th January I walked into the operating theatre. I was in surgery for ten hours while they put the electrodes in and spent two days in HDU and two weeks on the video telemetry ward before I underwent a second operation to remove the electrodes. During the first operation I lost two and a half pints of blood and had to have a blood transfusion whilst I was in HDU to replace the blood I lost. Pretty remarkable really, that the hospital managed to find blood to replace the blood I lost considering I have abnormal blood or a white cell deficiency.

After the operation I felt sick and had the most humungous headache ever and felt like karma had come along and bitten me on the back side. I was taken down to the high dependency unit where I was monitored. Up on recovery I was taken to the telemetry ward where the tests and investigations began. My medication was reduced and I was under observation for two weeks before a second operation took place to remove the electrodes.

The video EEG recorded up to nine seizures though I only recall two. I also had some weakness down my left side and it took me most of the first week to regain my strength. I found eating and drinking difficult and was sick for most of the two weeks that I was on the telemetry ward. It was after the first few days on the ward that the staff removed the drip and I was able to drink fluids by myself again. It took me ages to get out of the bed and on to a chair. I had to use bed pans, commodes, and have bed baths. I was taking anti sickness medication so that I could eat. I was unable to eat solids as my head hurt so much and felt so heavy, and I had to drink from a straw. The intracranial EEG also showed that I had a weak shoulder and during my time on the telemetry ward I also noticed that I had weakness down my left side. The weakness got stronger during the time I was in hospital; though I did have a small stroke of some sort whilst I was on the recovery ward during a visit to the toilet. The electrodes they put in were the size of credit cards and I was hooked up to a machine that monitored the electrical waves in the brain. Though I found the process rather interesting I felt like I done ten rounds in a boxing match and lost.

However I will never forgive the surgeons for sending my bra on a journey around the hospital in a kidney dish, I had never had an operation before so I didn't know I had to go down there in my birthday suit wearing nothing but a hospital gown. For the first week my bra sat there on the radiator in a kidney dish in my room and none of us knew it was there. No one would go near the kidney dish to investigate as we all thought it was medical responsibility and none of the staff knew what was in it. I had no idea what happened to my bra but was in too much pain during my first week to care.

It was a brave member of staff during my second week that chose to investigate the kidney dish and we both had a good laugh about it. Mystery solved about the missing bra anyway and a lesson learned for me. The idea of a surgeon removing my bra as well would any of you like that thought going through your mind?

During my second week on the telemetry ward I was starting to feel a bit more human and was finding I could hold down food and drink more easily. I was chattier and even up for doing a bit of research for the hospital. I was more mobile and watching TV, listening to my own music and writing again. I was even having a laugh and a joke with the staff.

I still found it difficult to get my head round the results of the various tests and come to a decision about further surgery. Though I was happy I had made the decision to go ahead with this intracranial surgery, I just wish it could have happened sooner. Perhaps if this kind of test was available to me as a teenager it would have helped me come to terms with my epilepsy back then. All the questions and struggles we went through could have been cut short. Mum was also finding coming to terms with my surgery difficult. I think she was in shock for the whole of the two weeks that I was in the telemetry unit. The worst part for her, was the risk and consequences of if I was to go ahead with further surgery.

My mum just switched off during the three years I spent undergoing medical investigations and visiting consultants at the London hospitals, because she could not deal with the reality of what I wanted. Mum felt that the surgery would make me worse and that it was too risky. She felt that having surgery would take away my independence and I would be taking away her independence too. There were quite a few arguments once I gave my consent and a lot of pressure on me not to go ahead with my decision.

By time it came round to having the intracranial or electrodes out I was feeling a lot better. I had the results from the tests and observations, and found that I now had a lot of questions answered and knew what my brain looked like. However, I was not liking what the professor was proposing or what I was hearing.

The operation to remove the intracranial took less time, but I was still in theatre for eight hours. Unlike the first operation when I walked down to theatre, this time I was taken down there in a wheel chair. Still the same rule applied, I sat myself on the theatre table and was alert to everything that took place right up to the surgeon inserting the drug that would knock me out and the oxygen mask I would wear for my breathing.

When I came round this time though I was in a recovery room, and would go straight onto a hospital ward as soon as there was a bed available for me.

My diagnosis was right temporal lobe focus with right occipital lobe atrophy. Main damage in the right half of my brain, with poor memory and visual spatial recall and weakness on my left side mainly in my right shoulder but since the intracranial EEG I was finding it was down the whole of my left side now.

The results also confirmed that I was partially sighted in my left side as well as having problems with my vision in both eyes. It would explain a lot from my childhood anyway.

So if I were to go on to have further surgery there would be a lot to consider; as I would be making a lot of sacrifices as well as the risks involved. There was left occipital lobe damage, complex partial seizures and depression. A lot to take in for anyone, although I was well aware of the damage to my brain and the riskI was taking, but I knew it was something I had to do. If I did not go ahead after all these years of searching then it would all be for nothing.

I was well aware of the risk to my vision and to my left side. Though my vision was screwed already in my opinion may be the operation would give us some answers. Besides it was a risk I was willing to take at the time if I would get some answers.

Also I was hoping that the answers would be simple and that the next phase would get easier. To be honest I never really thought about the risks, they were just obstacles if I thought over them too much. I been searching for an opportunity like this for some time now and now the time had come I was not about to allow anyone to talk me out of it.

I was told the investigation lead to loss of lots of blood, a Tia, **(mini stroke)** and weakness to my left side and both shoulders. My memory got worse and there was no definite cure with the split brain operation. I was devastated when I was told that the operation I'd had to put the probes in took ten hours and resulted in a blood transfusion. In order to take the probes out again took eight hours and I nearly died.

I accepted the surgical investigation and signed the consent form for the first operation, the intracranial EEG. I was happy and content with that although the results of the investigation were a lot to take in. Though I was informed in Scotland of fractures to my skull and some damage to the back of my brain I was not fully aware just how damaged my brain and skull were. I guess I only took it all in a few years down the line when I was re-investigated in London and I was once again told just how complicated my brain was. My emotional outburst was due to my frustration, lack of support from my mother and annoyance that there would be so much damage and sacrifice if I were to proceed. Although, it should be said that my mother was only trying to protect me as at the time I thought I could live without vision. I was hoping any further surgery would be straight forward. I was warned of left homonymous hemianopia and low risk of paralysis of the left arm and leg. After the first operation I discovered straight away that I experienced some kind of stroke and there was weakness to my left side. A small price to pay for an operation that would give me the answers I been searching for all my life. Plus I was also wishing for the chance of a further operation to become seizure free. This second operation carried further risk such has a second partial or small stroke, some problems with my vision which was clear and a difference in my pupils.

When I finally regained the use of both arms and legs and I managed to get out of the hospital I had a lot of thinking to do. I was very emotional as it was clear that the risks attached to the operation I wanted out-weighed my desire to go ahead. Although I really wanted this operation, something in the back of my mind was telling me I was better off the way I was. I knew that after having come all this way after doing years of research only to turn this operation down then I would spend my time in future working on other ways to reduce my seizures. I was now determined that there was some other way around this if surgical intervention was not a route I could take. First I needed to get my emotions under control since I had been struggling with depression for so long.

With the split brain operation the surgeon talked about there was a 50/ 50 chance of survival and I could lose my sight altogether. It would take another four years to recover from the intracranial video EEG, butat least I had some answers. I was told that I was born with a small skull and my brain got squashed at birth. It was the brain trauma or damage that could have caused the epilepsy. I was diagnosed with right temporal epilepsy with damage to the optical lobes. The proposal if I was to go ahead with the split brain operation was to split or remove the optical lobes. I was told this would leave me visually impaired but I did not need or require them. I figured the split brain was not worth it so withdrew from the proposal. I was devastated that it was not a cure. With a broken heart and tears in my eyes I decided not to go ahead.

Perhaps if the hospital had of turned me down due to the complications I might not have been such an emotional person since I would have known then that surgery was not for me. I would have been a stronger individual knowing that I could have just got on with my life taking on whatever I faced then. Perhaps then I would not have had people wrapping me up in cotton wool because they would have seen my strength and courage. However this procedure was not available to me back then as it was only available in the United States. I wish the option of going down the surgery route was available to teenagers and children when I was still going through my teens as I was continuously fighting with the hospital since no one was sure what my diagnosis was. I was fed up of been wrapped up in cotton wool and really at a time when a child needed to be a child I felt I was being protected and sheltered from anyone and everyone.

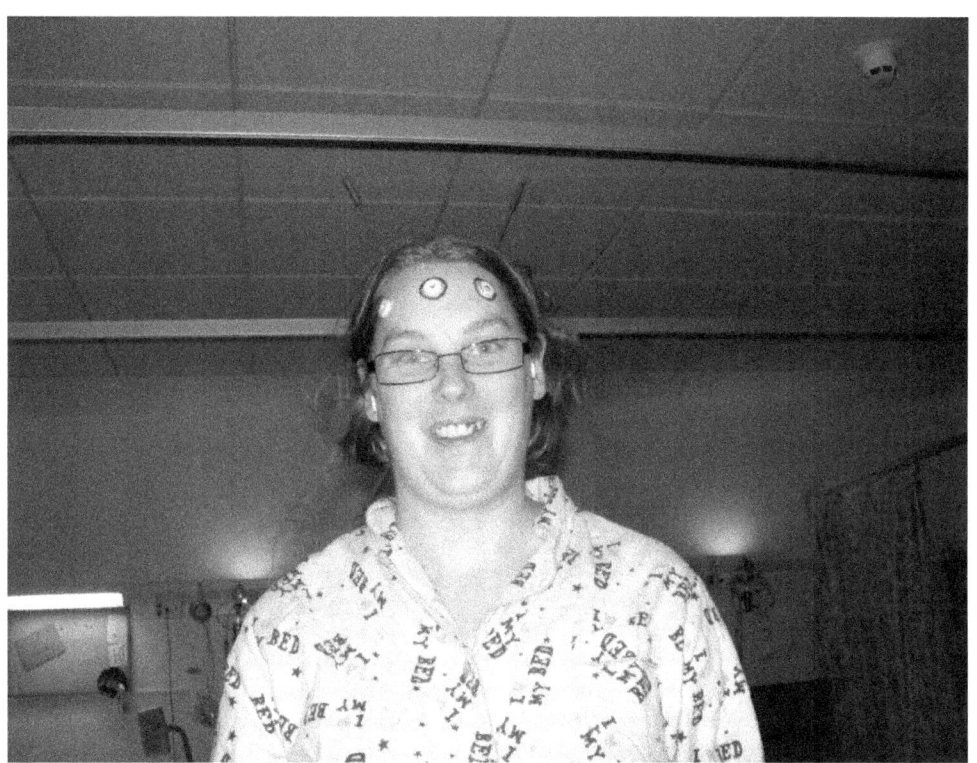

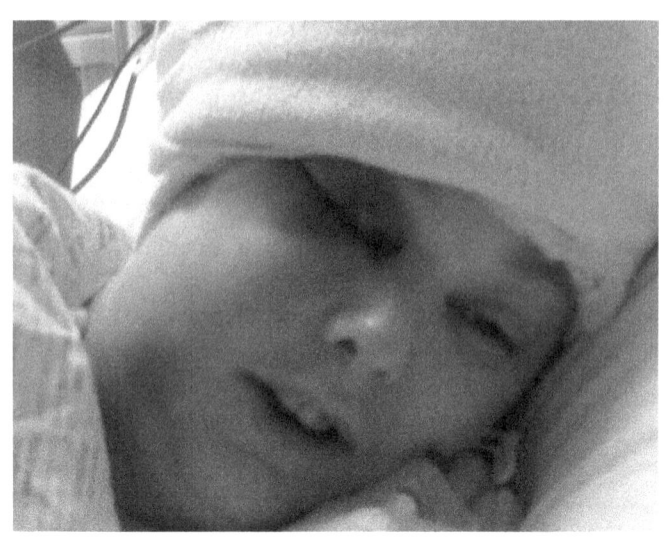

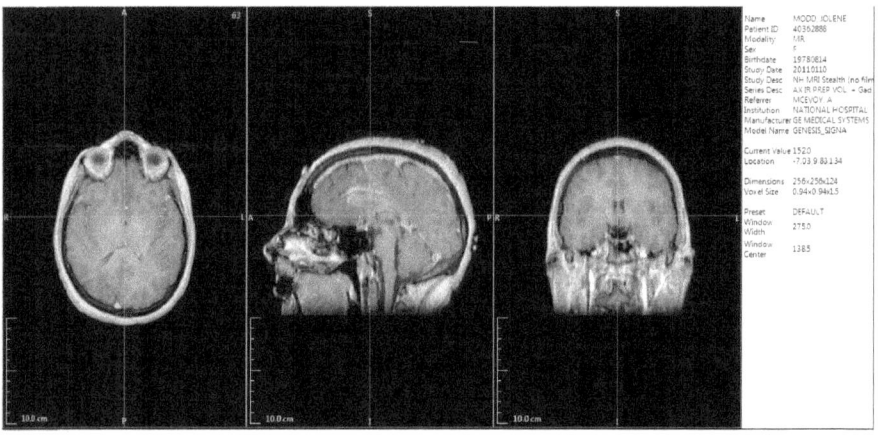

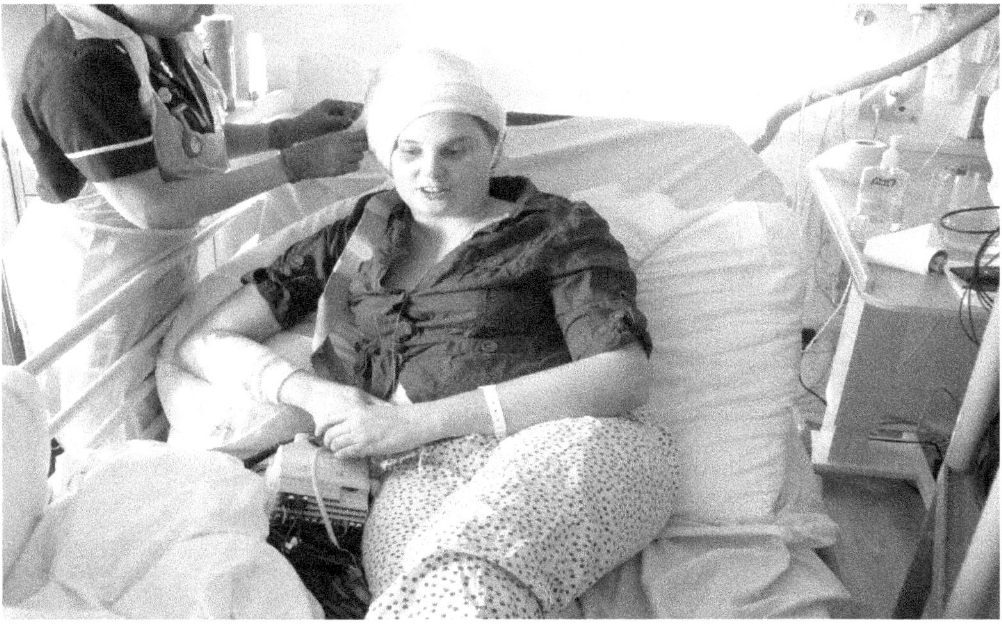

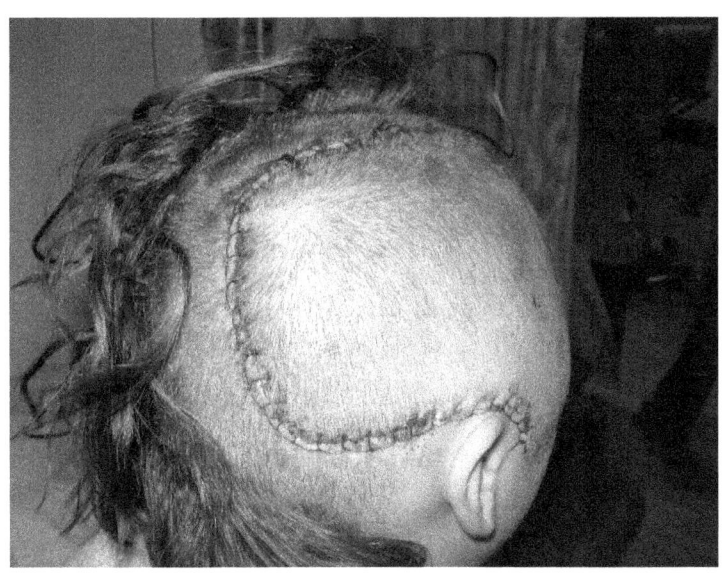

Chapter Thirteen

Recovery

The recovery from the investigation would be slow and taking in the information discovered through the operation would be stressful and emotional. I was not sure I was ready for what was coming my way. I finally found a consultant, professor and neuro surgeon who were offering me what I wanted. What I been waiting for and searching for this operation for the past ten years. Now I was about to turn it down which even to this day as I write still brings tears to my eyes, knowing that what I so wanted I could not have due to the high risk and sacrifices. I also knew I did not have the full support of my friends and family on my side. However I do not regret going through the investigation as it has answered many of my questions.

I checked out of hospital at the end of January and Mum came to stay with me for a few days until I was able to cope on my own. There were a few days when my legs would give way or I noticed my left hand wanted to do its own thing or would simply just not work.

I did wonder if I had one or two minor strokes or if it was simply weakness. The major difference I noticed was my vision. Often even with my glasses on, my left eye would experience double vision or I would often become sensitive to light. I found my eyes becoming tired more often and I was spending less time on the computer or reading. Since my eyes were becoming increasingly tired I found I was spending more time sleeping with little energy and less time doing the activities I enjoyed. The only time

I went outside was if I really had to. I don't really recall much of 2011. This was another reason for making the decision not to go ahead with the main operation.

Since reading and writing are two of my passions this was another reason for thinking a lot about my decision for further surgery, since I would lose my vision in my left side for certain. The risk of losing my sight in return for a one in three chance of becoming seizure free was something I was willing to consider at first. However, the more I tried to visualise my life without my sight the harder I found it to make my decision.

I would often experience shooting pains or spasms in my left hand which were new following the operation. I also noticed a difference to my little finger. It now felt like I had a dozen little plasters and bandages wrapped around it. There was a strange sensation in this finger for a good few months. At first the fingers on my left hand were not doing what they should be doing. Once they started to function and communicate I found that my little finger on my left hand would always remain separate. Occasionally I would feel a shooting pain or a coldness sensation, or pins and needles in that one finger. Other times that one finger would remain cold while the rest of my hand was warm. Then there were the pains in my head, on the side where I had my operation and I would often find myself massaging behind my ear then slowly working my hands or fingers up over the scar. For a while my head felt numb or spongy until I gained the sensations. Once the sensations came back I would often find parts of my head would feel sore or itchy. Sometimes there was one spot that felt as though there was fluid or lose bones although I could never locate the spot when it came to complaining to the doctor. I was never sure if it was in my head or part of the healing process or my soft spot. May be it was the part where the hospital inserted the drain. I could not get any answers about this from the support group websites, as if I ever asked a question other people were too busy asking questions themselves rather than supporting each other. So I would often refer to books or papers that had been published by doctors and consultants or pieces of research I could find on the internet.

Over the next few months my symptoms changed and I slowly recovered. I found myself getting back to normal and after a consultation with my neuro surgeon; turning down the offer of further surgery as I felt the risk were too high. I started college and continued to work on my books. I still had days where I relapsed and had seizures and I also continued to feel tired on a daily basis. I often experienced problems with sleep, suffering from insomnia, stress, anxiety and depression. I would go on to manage this in a range of ways.

Living with epilepsy has its problems. Managing it and living with it is a process we are forced to learn to live with. Medication, therapy and staying in contact with those who understand are all part of the process.

Chapter Fourteen

Research and Progress

In July 2011 I was discharged from the London hospitals and referred back to Salford and I made the decision at this point there was no further point in trying out anymore medication. I would stay at the dosage I was currently taking with Topiramate™ and allow my GP to take over my care. I also wanted to remain in contact with a specialist nurse in case I needed anyone to talk to or had any concerns. Although Topiramate™ had its side effects I was able to manage this myself by changing my diet and way of life, however some side effects remained.

I had spent years going round in circles and as far as I was concerned I had **no intention** of continuing on that journey. I had turned down the VNS (Vagus Nerve Stimulator/ Implant) because I lived alone and was still on medication. I continued to do my own research as I recovered at home.

I discovered two other names for the other symptoms I was experiencing since the neurosurgery but as a spiritual person who also believes in alternative therapies and being a little philosophical I wanted to look a little deeper before I was willing to accept any more labels or communicate my new symptoms to the doctors.

I had an appointment with my epilepsy specialist nurse and neuro psychiatrist in January so I had time to do further research before approaching either one with my latest symptoms. I found most of the neuro science and brain books or epilepsy books made a lot of sense however spiritual books and psychology books seemed to share a lot in common also. There were a lot of documentaries that seemed to have their roots in neurosurgery which made me wonder why my neurologist never took me seriously in the past.

The neuro science books contained a lot of language and terminology that was often too technical to understand although I could understand enough to see that I had encountered a lot of nerve damage from the neuro surgery which would explain why my left hand did not function in the same way when typing and carrying objects or lifting. My left arm is a lot weaker since neuro surgery and my left hand often behaves like it is dyslexic. Also from what I could understand there was some visual damage in my right temporal lobe or right side that had affected my left eye. I now sometimes encounter some double vision in my left eye from time to time.

I also wondered about how the surgery had affected my motor cortex has I had never encountered the spongy feeling before surgery. There had been the odd occasion over the years where I had encountered the big head or **Alice in Wonderland Syndrome**. This would seem as though the room went all weird and my head felt huge whilst I was sitting down; or the room becoming brighter or larger or smaller and I panicked during this time. There were a few times when this happened and I was unable to find the door to get out of the room. Over the years I often felt I had these seizures in my sleep as though I was dreaming them, or the seizures would occur up on waking. I would wake up and find the room would look distorted. Doctors, consultants and neurologist all put this experience down to just another seizure although I did not always encounter a seizure; sometimes I just encountered a migraine or felt a little tired.

Sometimes I would go for ages without any occurring and not always associate the migraine attacks and tiredness with the seizures which was often frustrating. Especially, when I was never sure if the migraine attacks and seizures were related to each other or if either were a sign that I was going to have a bad day. I got to the stage when I stopped waiting for the seizures to happen. Epilepsy was controlling my life and my anxiety was just getting worse.

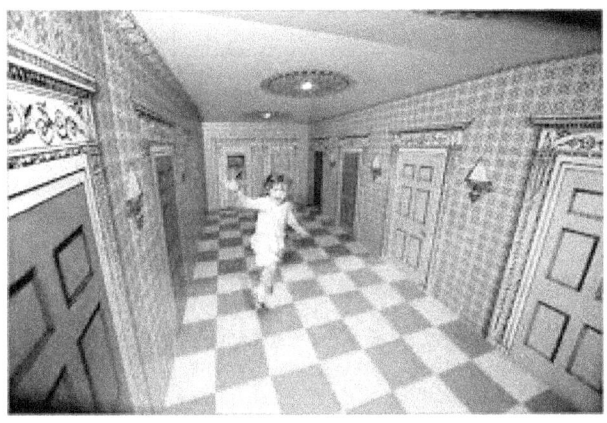

In terms of my vision after the intracranial EEG I was told I had a partial blindness in my left eye. This would explain the problems I have had with my vision all my life. I often see the street lights as spectacular light shows; glowing and joining each other in the street. Often I can see this not just with street lights but car lights and sometimes torches and general house lights all look to me like fog lights. I have never been bothered by these spectacular light shows as to me this is normal; however I now understand the way in which I perceive light is due to a combination of my partial blindness in the left eye and short sightedness.

I discovered that the visual problems are at the back of the brain in the cortex. I also researched vitamin deficiency, diet and depression although I would wait until after my appointments with the doctors and until I had relocated before looking into diet and vitamin deficiencies properly.

The first thing I had to sort out was my depression; I had tried anti-depressants in the past even prior to surgery though none so far had agreed with my system. Antidepressants seemed to interact with my antiepileptic medication or seizures or make my stress worse. The buzzing sound in my head had now gone along with the strange thoughts or feelings; however I knew I was still feeling depressed and emotional. I was no longer hearing the repeat noises or echoing sounds that I experienced back in 2010 when I felt I was having a psychological break down. At that point I was not too sure if it was the antidepressants or stress I was experiencing from the emotional disturbances or build-up of stress from the hospital in London. I hated travelling on a train or the sound of children at that point as the sound stayed with me long after the train had departed or I had left the station. Even after a child had left the supermarket I could still hear them. If my boyfriend woke me up snoring I could hear noises that were not there for a long time after. My only release was listening to music through head phones.

Now, not having to go through the stress of hospitals I wondered if I could give the antidepressants another go. I wondered if I could find the right one for me. This time I might have a different experience. All I had to do now was make an appointment with my GP. In the mean time I would return to my research and my books. I also bought some vitamin supplements whilst waiting for my appointments with various doctors.

I found myself adjusting my diet to supplement the vitamins I was deficient in which helped a lot of the side effects I encountered with the medication I was on for my epilepsy. Though none of which helped with my depression.

I tried out suggested diets and cutting out various foods such as broccoli, oranges and lemons, citrus fruits such as grape fruit, drinks that are high in caffeine such as coffee and cola, fizzy drinks and alcohol. I replaced white bread and rice and some spicy foods with brown pasta and rice and whole meal brown bread. All of the foods on the list that I was to cut out unfortunately were amongst my favourite however I did not mind removing alcohol as I did not miss this. It would take some time before I found the balance of replacing my vitamin supplements with food and finding a cure for my depression through food or eating my way to healthy wellbeing I found I was sleeping a lot and constantly feeling tired.

I replaced sugar with honey and started shopping in the "free from" range. I used soya free products and goat's milk when cooking and bought some vitamin and mineral books and low calorie and low fat or fat free cooking books. My intention was not to go on a diet but to use the books as a guide to help me to cook healthier meals. I wanted to cook and prepare food that was better for me. Regardless of the blood test results I'd had that confirmed I was low in calcium and other vitamins; my consultants and doctors all felt my blood results were fine even though it did not counter out the tiredness, nose bleeds or other symptoms. I hoped that if this was the case the new diet I was on might improve my blood results. I wanted to replace the vitamins that I had lost according to the results I had seen and books I had read that would help improve my immune system and heal my body. The aim was to eat foods rich in protein that the body was not producing. By changing the way I ate I hoped to improve my depression and reduce my seizures and stress. What I did not realise is that I was doing a diet that already existed that had already been done before and I was simply repeating history.

I started to focus more on what new members on the forums were saying. I found that these new members were now following in my footsteps but this time they were bringing my attention back to the research I had done when I started college.

The **Glutamate Aspartate Restricted Diet** consists of cutting out gluten, dairy products, corn and soya which are the four main triggers of epilepsy. Wheat, yeast and gluten are the main three triggers of depression. It was a few months after sticking to this diet that I found my seizures reduced and I started to feel an improvement with my depression.

It was pretty clear I was still recovering from the neurosurgery that I'd had the year before. I had heard that recovery could take a few years, although me being me, I was expecting to be up and running after my first year. Conversations with friends who had been through neurosurgery spoke about how fatigued they also felt for one or two years afterwards.

I lost a lot of weight although my weight loss was not down to stress or anxiety it was due to my healthier lifestyle. I felt I was being affected by a combination of things; change of diet, stress, change in weather conditions, my immune system and my neutropenia. I made some enquires with my

132

dietician and epilepsy specialist although they did not seem that concerned and further enquires at my doctors insisted it might be the weather or my medication.

I was now feeling safer and more at ease in my new flat but even so depression and seizures were still a problem and part of my life. Taking daily vitamins, using crystals and colour therapy and watching comedy shows did ease my depression.

A diet of fish, chicken and liver seemed to be working for me. I was eating more brown rice than pasta and eating more fresh fruit and vegetables. My sleep had improved but I still experienced a lot of tiredness. In addition, moving to a new area meant I was spending a lot of time on the computer but was not going anywhere or doing anything. I really feel that regardless of who you are, or whatever your disability may be, it is important to socialise and meet people. In order to treat a condition it is important to look at the whole situation. What is the point in talking about something or treating it with a pill if you're not going to treat the whole situation?

It was months after, I was introduced to a nutritionist who reminded me of a diet which now had a name to it. It was called the **FODMAP diet** which was basically what I had been doing only it involved cutting out even more of the foods that were causing my symptoms and slowly re-introducing the foods over a short period of time to find the triggers of my food intolerance or possible allergies that could be linked to my condition. I found that by cutting out all the food I enjoyed not only did I relieve the feeling of nausea but I also eased the stomach pains and reduced the amount of seizures I encountered or experienced every month. I also managed to reduce the amount of anxiety I experienced and ease my depression although I still experienced fatigue. Coffee, chocolate and sugar seemed to trigger off nausea and also affected my sleep.

I discovered that amino acids are very important in the correct functioning of the brain. A generalized deficiency in them can lead to symptoms such as apathy, concentration difficulties, and loss of interest, insomnia, mood swings, anxiety, depression, self-mutilation and aggression. I started my research into amino acids in 2007 and started consciously practicing this diet in 2012. My nutritionist introduced me to "taurine", a supplement which is an amino acid. I started to add these to my diet whilst shopping in the "free from" section. I found that over time my seizures reduced and my depression improved though the seizures did raise some concern with some of the locals living in the area. Given the fact that I was required to get work I did wonder how I would face this next challenge.

I actually found through the FODMAP diet that I could tolerate soya and would often make use of soya products. I also replaced cow's milk with goat's milk and started taking vitamin supplements and calcium supplements. I was also not having as many nose bleeds since I increased my vitamin c supplements. My nose bleeds were only present when my immune system was low, I been lying down, the temperature of the room was too high, I missed my medication, first thing in the morning and late at night or during my menstrual cycle. I would increase my vitamin c and d during this time. However as much as I had managed to reduce my depression and seizures through changing my diet I felt my fatigue and tiredness was more anxiety and stress related and would not benefit from diet alone. I needed to embark on the stress and anxiety course once more.

The stress and anxiety management course did help me manage to do my shopping and helped with social interaction but I found in terms of my epilepsy it did nothing for my depression. Especially since my depression and epilepsy were linked. However, trying to combat depression and epilepsy through diet and medication was hard. I found that as they were linked I felt that I was fighting a losing battle since most of the research I did got published through other means by other professors and doctors I did not know. Often when browsing the web I would find out if any of my research was useful or a success.

In 2013, although I had already completed a stress and anxiety course and qualified in stress and anxiety management back in 2000; I found myself once more enrolling on the same course but this time with a bit of a twist. I was now doing this course for therapeutic purposes. I felt that my symptoms could be a number of different things; however doctors had told me I did not have I.B.S, was not gluten intolerant and I was not a celiac or diabetic. I had all the symptoms of these conditions and could not lose weight around my stomach. I was feeling constantly sick after consuming dairy products and eating certain foods. I had looked into food intolerance, cutting out gluten and changing my diet for depression. Yet all the symptoms were rooted with my anxiety. I was still feeling tired and fatigued but in order to follow my ambition and turn my hobby into a career I first needed to get these symptoms under control.

In 2013 I decided to take the **FODMAP diet** very seriously and began to keep a diary of what I ate, how many seizures I had each month, when they started and how I felt. I found that my body rejected almost everything I ate and I had to go back to bland basic food.

Since I had surgery there has been a lot of research published in the press, including more awareness that has reminded me of information given to me over the years by the professors, doctors and neurologists I've come into contact with. The same information is used for rugby players, research linked to dementia and brain injuries. Whenever I make queries or ask charities questions these days I am usually accused of worrying so I only ever write about it in my poetry and books. I was always told about the lack of oxygen to the brain. Being a tall person, I was always told to squat or bend over and was told about diet, certain foods that could block the digestive system or starve the body of oxygen. Drinking plenty of fluids, and eating the right foods, is important especially around hormonal periods, such as the menstrual cycle. Keeping hydrated, getting the right amount of sleep and having the right amount of sun.

I mentioned earlier in my story, my mother's frustration with medical establishments and staff. There are still mothers out there that feel this frustration for their own children and often this frustration and anxiety is passed on to the doctors or consultants who are the first point of call when a mother or patient is angry or frustrated with their condition or care.

However, some things today are done differently. I have worked with a range of services and organisations to campaign for people with disabilities to be treated equally. I find consultants and doctors will now work *with* you and communicate with patients and carers a lot more than they used to. There are also a lot more organisations and charities to provide help and support to families and carers. I have found that there is a lot more information available on the internet, a wider availability of books, and more support groups. All of this has helped to relieve a lot of my own anxiety and help my mental state. The more I have used these services the less stressed I have been myself, and this has helped to control my seizures.

Mental health and depression is part and parcel of epilepsy, the more seizures a person has, the more likely they are to suffer from depression.

It was much worse when I was a child and throughout my teens. I was always told I was an emotional child and often told to snap out of it. Apparently back then children did not suffer from depression or anxiety. These conditions did not exist in a child. I recall my nursery teacher shaking me because I could not find my coat. My mother walked in on her shaking me as I was crying my eyes out. I was simply informed that I was an emotional child with whom the stigma and labels stuck until the day I left school.

Being told you are soft or "emotional" does nothing for a child's self-esteem or confidence. Not much was understood about epilepsy and patient/doctor relationships were not as they are now. There were still arguments going on about my diagnoses and what types of seizures I was having and if they were at all seizures or fits. No one really compared the two or recognised the difference between attacks of fainting or giddiness, panic attacks, anxiety attacks or epilepsy in general.

I actually found such conditions difficult to prove even in my early twenties. I found I had to go to college and study or research such conditions in order to get a diagnosis during the nineties. Research has shown that tiredness, insomnia and a weak immune system is all part of depression; especially depression related to sleep disorders and long term medical conditions.

I now had the opportunity to sort out my health whilst doing the research and concentrating on my books. I would also have the opportunity to set up a business and work for myself.

I could use my research and the support groups to help raise awareness and my time to get more involved in the many campaigns I had previously been involved in. So, I became more accepting of my life and my condition and started to focus more on raising awareness and educating others.

If I got too tired or over excited, stressed or anxious then it was likely that I would have seizures. I found I was able to reduce my seizures by introducing vitamin c and zinc into my diet. I started taking amino acids or protein supplements and changed my diet.

Over a period of months my seizures reduced from 25 seizures a month to 11 seizures a month. The main cluster of seizures occurred during my menstrual cycle. I found that sudden changes in temperature and stress also triggered my seizures. My occupational therapist stayed with me for the first year whilst I moved in to the new flat until I settled in.

Chapter Fifteen

Family Reunions

On June the 5th 2013 my grandfather passed away after spending weeks in hospital. I never got to know my granddad properly. I recall chatting to him sometimes on Salford precinct when I was a teenager before his memory started to decline. When my grandparents moved on to the estate I grew up and we moved away. I used to visit my grandparents when I was a teenager when I hung around with my cousins whilst still at school. Back then I felt that I was part of the family and it never really bothered me that I did not know my father or my brothers or sisters.

I come from two large families, on my father's side my epilepsy is evident. My grandfather and a number of cousins have a diagnosis of epilepsy. Although I did not meet my father until I was fifteen, I was always brought up to be aware of my father and his side of the family. It made little difference to me that both my mother and father had a large family. The fact that they knew who I was, was enough. It made no difference that epilepsy ran in my father's side of the family. I still felt like an outcast. My grandfather on my dad's side was also no closer to me. though i have memories of him welcoming me into the family when he was alive.

My siblings and my father however, still claimed I was not related despite having obvious proof and a DNA test done when I was a baby. However once my cousin passed me the phone number which contained the contact for my father everything changed. I have no regrets meeting my father, and getting to know my family. There are plenty of children out there who never get that chance.

I know who I am and where I came from as a result. Meeting my father at the age of fifteen as completed me.

On my father's side of the family there is also a history of ADD, depression, Muscular dystrophy, problems with the blood and other disabilities. I got to know the various members of my family as I grew up and throughout my school days although I was never close to any of them. Although despite spending four years with my father I never made a connection with him or my siblings. Eventually we went our separate ways though I stayed in touch with one of my cousins whom I went to school with and grew up with. I found that I was closer to my cousin than any other member of my family. I was actually hurt when she settled down with her first sun as I felt I had lost that connection.

As we both grew up and my cousin settled down and had children we both went our separate ways. I did eventually resume my connection with my cousin when I found her again through a social networking site. She was now living round the corner from her mum and younger brother so I went round to see them whenever I could. As my younger cousin's muscular dystrophy deteriorated I found I went round less but I was able to keep in touch with the whole family with the use of the internet.

My cousin and her brothers and sisters were all now married with children and I went round when I could, but I was not as close to the family as I once was during school and college.

I sometimes went to various family events but found myself feeling left out and distant. I found that I often accepted the isolation and my own company. I kept in touch with my cousins and members of my family online through Facebook. Occasionally I would go round, although isolation became part of my life over the years. it became a great benefit to me whilst working on and writing my books.

Once I decided I was never going to have a relationship with my siblings I tried again with my father without my brothers and sisters around. I attended one of my cousins fundraising events in the hope I could sell a few books and support my cousin's charity at the same time and reconnect with the family. However my father left the room. I think he felt uncomfortable, I found myself trying too hard to fit in and socialise with people who were strangers to me. Even though I knew a lot of them from school and through Facebook it was harder to reconnect this time. I once again felt alone in a room full of people I knew. I was invited to a few events after the one I attended but I never felt part of the family after that event.

I went to a wellbeing fair with my mother where I had a reading and my granddad came through. When I had learned that my granddad was ill and in hospital, although I wanted to visit him I found going down too difficult even when I was in the area. At the moment I heard my granddad had passed away I felt a bit emotional; but as the day progressed I found I felt no emotions what's so ever. I had no compulsion to talk about it or share the news with anyone. I never knew my granddad and never felt I was close or part of the family. All of my siblings and my father told me I had to take a second DNA test to prove I was my father's child and even then I was told I would have to pay for it. Yet my father was willing to give me thousands of pounds each year for birthdays and Christmas while I was in his life.

I was introduced to his family and everyone knew about me yet he rejected me because his mother did not approve. I would have been a daddy's girl growing up as I always wanted my daddy. I have always been emotional and given the fact that my granddad died having had a diagnosis of epilepsy, I will never understand my father and my father's side of the family.

When it came to my mother's side of family life was even more complicated. My family each had too many of their own issues to be concerned with mine. They may have been close as I was growing up but as they were only half related each had emotional battles to deal with. The family was full of emotional and physical disability so had a lot of psychological healing to deal with.

In May 2013 my mother paid my grandmother a visit. Of course I was there for moral support. I understood the family and their issues but I left each of them to go their own way. Of course I spoke to each of them and accepted each member of my family and their issues. Unlike my father's side of the family when I felt like the outsider; I was more like the counselling service when it came to my mother's side of the family. I rarely heard from anyone until they had something they wanted to get of their chest or they were in trouble. It was actually hard to believe that I was the one who needed the support. It was more mental health, anxiety disorder, depression and learning disability that was evident in my mother's side of the family. My mother's side of the family had problems with communication, understanding themselves, personal development, dyslexia and developmental problems. Due to these problems my family were too busy being distracted with their own issues that they were not aware of what was going on around them. When something did go wrong in the family they were there for each other but often the problem had got so bad that they got there too late for any of them to do something about it. I hoped that I was able to reach the younger generation as the elders seemed to be learning about themselves and life a little too late. What I found however, was that the new generation of cousins were now making the same mistakes whilst crying about the same issues. It was now time for me and my mother to step in and try and do something about it. Now that my uncles were now starting to understand life I wondered if it was now time for a family reunion.

The problem was there was too much bitterness and lack of understanding in the family. I had many family members come to me but I was unsure if any of them were willing to sit and listen.

How could I overcome such an obstacle? I could go weeks without hearing from a family member and given my epilepsy I wondered why no one was concerned. When I thought about the illness in my family and why they ignored each other until they themselves had a problem they wanted resolving. Why were we not closer?

I would see my mum once a week for bingo but if I had a seizure whilst I was with her she would panic. Yet I thought my mum understood my condition but she treated me like a child or like I was disabled. It was an issue I wanted to get to the bottom of but I too struggle to understand my mother and my mother's family. Then again this was a similar ignorance and behaviour that I experienced in a work setting and by society. The year was 2015 and I was starting to feel like we had gone backwards in time.

My mother's family are not close themselves. My mother did not grow up with her family and did not get to know all her family until she was older. My mother was fostered out and her two brothers and sister were split up. When she was eventually reunited they were teenagers. My mother being the youngest did not feel she got to know her siblings that well, therefore my mother also feels like a stranger when surrounded by her siblings. This often makes it difficult for me when I want to spend time with my mother's family because I feel like I do not know them. So getting to know my mother's family again was a big deal for us all.

In February 2013 I put myself up for election on the Epilepsy Action Committee Members Board and then found that in May 2013 I was put up for election. It was a step up for me as I was able to make a difference. My research with the hospitals was also making an impact and I was also making progress with my books. Though my granddad did not think that voluntary work was acceptable, He found it difficult to accept that there was no paid work out there for me. He also had a hard time taking self-employment seriously. I however felt I was making progress. My next step was to challenge the job centre on my next meeting.

My mother was building bridges with her siblings, I was getting to know my cousins and my mother's family was slowly coming together again. I was also in touch with other members of the family though I knew this would be a slow process given the history.

Epilepsy is not a learning disability or mental health condition, although there is a psychological factor involved, although this did not occur until my condition presented its self in some way.

I have epilepsy so why treat me any differently to a person in a wheel chair or a person who has depression? I regularly post and blog about epilepsy and other conditions in order to raise awareness although I often find not many people will respond. When I first started blogging and using the internet as a tool I had a lot of followers and fans who would respond to and like my posts. These days I am lucky to get one share.

Chapter Sixteen

Living with Epilepsy and the Perceptions of Others

I've found that I have suffered with short term memory function and have had difficulty recalling aspects of 2011 onwards.

I am aware of the fatigue, tiredness, IBS symptoms and other side effects of the medication that must frustrate those around me when I do my best to contribute. I see other people's frustration not that I feel they always understand how I am feeling. I have been on both ends of the spectrum. The medication I take now is only a low dosage but it still affects me to the annoyance of those around me. I have been drugged up and spaced out a lot more than I am now and often meet people who are that spaced out it takes them a good few hours to get going. I can see why my mother was so frustrated and why others around me find it easier just to refuse to employ me or avoid me completely. Just understanding the frustration I see the reason for the avoidance and ignorance.

It was so much harder for me to get work whilst on medication than it was off medication. There is always the debate that goes through my mind. Do I go for the treatment and accept the ignorance, misunderstanding, avoidance, loneliness and isolation for having a medical condition I was born with? Or do I ignore the treatment and risk the life and concern of others just so that I can have a social life, friends and acceptance from others? I can see why a lot of people with diagnoses of epilepsy prefer to die young and refuse treatment rather than go through the stress of finding the right medication. At least if they ignore the risk they might be accepted by society.

I enjoyed most of my employment and if only circumstances were right or I was not moving on or relocating then I would have happily stayed at some of the places where I had worked. I tried everything I could think of to keep hold of my job till eventually pressure and stress took its toll and I gave in. Over the years I found myself signing on and off job seekers though I only ever looked at this as temporary or short term. It has always remained an ambition of mine to become self-employed one day and not to let my medical condition get in the way.

Though I do like my own independence and have always enjoyed having my own place, having epilepsy can also be isolating. However, sometimes the thought of depending on someone else to come into your life to cook, clean or assist you in anything else can also be seen as an intrusion. I understand why a person with epilepsy sometimes pushes that sort of help away. Though I sometimes would love some help there is always that part of me that feels like my independence is being stolen. It is the same when it comes to applying for work.

I know I have a lot to offer society but when someone turns me away on the grounds of my epilepsy I feel like I am been sent a message that I am useless and have nothing to offer. All of which has an effect on my confidence and anxiety; and while I might say to myself I am not that bothered I am aware of the psychological implication this has had on me.

The government have never passed a bill that many charities have campaigned for when running the Campaign for Change. The government's argument is that we can have a seizure anywhere which is true of course. I have had seizures in places that would give you nightmares. The scariest ones have always occurred in the front seats of cars which often meant the driver pulling over onto the hard shoulder on the motorway. I have also been in a friend's car in which the driver crashed the car upon witnessing my seizure. I realise just how frightening my seizures can be and just how dangerous they can be also.

When I came out of work in 2008 I got more involved in charities as I wanted to raise awareness. I had two motives really; one it was too easy to go back on benefits and I felt the job centre did not do enough to help me get another job when I came out of work. The second was the stigma and ignorance I was noticing when I came out of work. I suddenly found myself unemployable and worse still treated like some crazy person who should be locked up. The more I campaigned the more horror stories I heard. So I wanted people to see just how independent I was and just how intelligent I was. I was not ill. I had a medical condition that perhaps limited me to some things in life but it did not affect me or stop me from living with this condition or having a life. At this time there were networks out there I could use on the internet for support and to talk to others but social networking sites like Twitter MySpace and Facebook opened up plenty of opportunities for me.

I campaigned for more specialist counsellors to be in place, as I felt that not all counsellors fully understood the vast amount of medical conditions; and this often made therapy difficult. I found myself studying psychology, counselling and other therapy techniques to enable me to get a better understanding of therapy and the mind. I would go to **AGM** meetings to talk to therapists and hospital staff about therapy and epilepsy and other conditions so that I could get this message across. Eventually my local hospital put in a neuro psychiatrist to specialise in this particular area.

I never allow my condition to get to me. I keep myself busy and always find something to do.

When I am having a bad day I use my microwave or electric steamer to cook, for safety reasons so that I am not having the fire brigade coming out to me. There are various safety precautions that can be put in place to ensure safety when a person is in seizure mode. It also helps to keep the neighbours and family members informed if you plan to go away or go out for the day.

When I feel too rough to chance the bath I either do my hair in the sink or go to the hair dressers. I have a wash down or I stay in bed and rest. I simply take my time. I can do my shopping online or go into the store and get it delivered. If I am feeling energetic I bring the shopping back myself or mum comes over and we go shopping together. If I am really bad there really is no need to leave the flat. I can do everything online and even order my food if I can't microwave it. I cook, I clean and do everything myself as much as I can. If I have a seizure in the house my main concern is that no one will know about it so if I am feeling rough I stay on the sofa or stay in bed. I have had friends in the past who have passed away who had epilepsy.

A friend once compared epilepsy to dying. He said you don't remember being born or being brought into this world just like you don't remember leaving. During a seizure he does not always have a strange feeling, or Deja-vu. He told me his perception does not change, his seizure comes on him too fast that he has no time to do anything about it or tell anyone.

Interesting that the cause of death for my two friends was sudden unexplained death or they died from their injuries. Since they lived on their own I had no idea how long it was before they were found or if they managed to press their helpline or emergency call button if they had one. That is my main worry since there are a lot of single people out there living with epilepsy who do not always require medical assistance in a way that they need to go to hospital every time they have a seizure but it's that one fatal time when they have that one attack that could be the life or death situation. Not everyone has that support or back up from family or friends or their next door neighbour when they live on their own. This has always stuck in my mind, every time I have had a seizure living on my own but I always want to maintain my independence. I am not afraid of death. It is the thought of not being found or how long it might take before someone found me; considering the amount of people that now live on their own.

I love my independence and living on my own and I have even got used to the idea of living with epilepsy and the fact that I have to accept that an operation may not be suitable for me. I have now accepted my condition now though it has taken me a long time. I will go out on my own even on one of the days when I am feeling anxious or having a partial seizure, or not feeling grounded. Life goes on, and there is not always another person upon which to rely. It could have been worse; I could have chosen the split brain operation and spent 2012 in hospital going through rehab having to learn how to live again. Rather than sitting here at the computer writing this book.

When I am feeling a little queasy and my feet do not want to work or do not feel connected to the ground I still do my best to get on with my life, make my tea or go to the shop.

After I was attacked outside a block of flats I lived in by a drug addict whilst recovering from neuro surgery I decided to move down south. I eventually settled into a ground floor flat in a small town in the middle of the country side. The town is friendly and supportive though I learned various ways of protecting myself and keeping myself safe. Having epilepsy can make a person very vulnerable at times, I have gone through a great deal, and now understand how to manage risk such as using the microwave or electric streamer instead of a cooker, having a shower instead of a bath, living on the ground floor and using a ruck sack and hand bag with a long strap so that it can't be stolen or lost in the event of a seizure. It has meant only carrying the amount of money I need and keeping my keys on a key ring that can be attached to my bag or a safe place. I have found that over the years the seizures, black outs and fainting attacks I have had have made me an easy target for muggings, and other attacks. So keeping my valuables safe and ensuring I do not become an easy target for thieves is essential. Even if that means spending a fortune on taxis to reach my destination.

I lock my front door regardless of whether I am in or out. I also make use of a bum bag which is much easier than a hand bag. The problem with fainting or blacking out is when coming round from these attacks a person can become easily confused and leave their hand bag or ruck sack unattended. So I take small steps when I am out and about. It is ideal to carry a mobile phone although I need to make sure I have a good signal, most countryside areas don't have good network coverage. I used to advise people to carry medical identification with them although now it is illegal to go into another person's bag or wallet unless you work for the police or another emergency service. So to have the identification in the form of a bracelet is more appropriate. Also if I am travelling alone I ensure that I carry my medication and identification with me.

I've done a lot of this although I am sure most people will ring the emergency services anyway and although I still find this rather annoying in a work setting it is something I am used to. It also helps to be first aid and epilepsy awareness trained or to carry something with you to this effect. If you can, find out if your organisation, employer or the people you work with have some first aid training and find out who they are.

Moving into the ground floor flat with a shower meant I was also closer to my mum and was able to concentrate on my books. However moving out of the city and into a small town did have its teething problems.

Epilepsy is a common condition though it is clearly one of the most misunderstood conditions and one of the most stigmatised. Probably almost everyone will come into contact with someone or know someone who has epilepsy.

Regardless the fears and stigmas still stick and dominate - even the mention of the word. That is before the vision of a person dropping down and shaking with eyes and head turning like something out of the exorcist. So for me moving from a city to a small town would be like putting a fish into a small fish tank. It would only take a few seizures and the whole town would know me. With my poor visual memory and inability to recall faces and names I would probably be known as the ignorant one. Quite often I have noticed that having a short term memory over the years has got me into trouble. As a child I was often accused of lying and telling tales because people did not understand my short term memory. I also noticed as I got older the accusation changed and I was often told I was confused or perceived as stupid; or treated like I was some kind of idiot.

This could explain why so many people who are ignorant to epilepsy see people like me as some kind of demon or freak; or simply do not want to entertain me.

People have perceived me as a mad woman who ought to be locked up somewhere safe who is on drink or drugs. Some of my seizures were described in this way "a drunken woman". If I was with a partner then they would probably be blamed for the bruises.

On the one hand my mother and family members assume that I need looking after and on the other, the government are saying I have to work because I am capable of working; this is an example of the conflicting information that I often hear from people who do not understand. Often some of the assumptions I experience can lead to a mix of over anxious people or total avoidance. The anxiety being the assumption that I cannot look after myself and the avoidance being the assumption that I am ok and there is nothing wrong with me.

People react differently to a person having a seizure. Paramedics were begging me to go home and stay at home, or to go to the hospital to be supervised overnight. Then there are those that assume I am a diabetic which at one point because I have a lot of symptoms which are very similar to a diabetic I actually started to think that perhaps I also had diabetes. Then there are those who over react and think I should be supervised at all times and should have someone do my cooking, cleaning and shopping as I could not possibly be capable of doing any of the above.

My perception changes just before a seizure. I get a strange feeling in the body and a sense of panic which might explain my strange behaviour to the observer or witness. If it is a partial seizure it could be a strange taste or smell that can last all day or for minutes. Sometimes I get a headache or migraine; regardless the experience can be overwhelming.

Not many people will talk openly about epilepsy or even offer to help or assist during a seizure. However this is the silent disability that I have been given. If I was to pass out or fall down then there is nothing I can do about it. The best a person can do is to put me in the recovery position and to call an ambulance and stay with me until the ambulance arrives.

I did happen to have a seizure in a local supermarket once and while the supermarket were very supportive, patient with me and knowledgeable it took me a while before I managed to get over my own embarrassment to go back to the same shop. I found that attitudes have changed in a lot of places but there were a lot of places where I found I was still uncomfortable. A friend of mine found that certain shops and supermarkets that were experienced and knowledgeable in health and safety and first aid seemed to do better in business than shops and stores that seemed to discriminate against people with disability. Is epilepsy so feared and stigmatised that people are too afraid to be seen with someone or is anyone who lives on their own these days associated with such a label that they might be deemed as a weirdo or psycho? Have we entered a society in which it is classed as too dangerous now to enter someone's house or check on a person on the street for fear of our own safety?

Up until 2000 years ago it was thought that epilepsy was linked to demons and gods and people were actually locked away, shunned and tortured. If I were an animal I would be put down. Unfortunately attitudes have not changed even in this century. The only difference being that spiritualism is more acceptable and that doctors and surgeons are more willing to work with their patients and vice versa.

There are more of us living in the community and living on our own with the help of charities, support workers and social workers. Asylums and institutions closed down back in the 1970s leaving only modern organisations which were opened up in order to give people a break and assistance to us with the means of support. With the help of nurses and doctors I was able to enjoy a life of independence and get the support I needed. Although it may have only been information and I had to wait for the internet and the help and advice from charities I was happier that my

155

relationship with the doctors and epilepsy specialist was improving. I did get an assessment from a social worker and an occupational health eventually, although unfortunately I did not meet the category needed for extra support. When I did eventually have an O.T come to visit me it was difficult to arrange support. I had a shower stool and chair delivered and was put in touch with a support worker. Though it was rather difficult to establish support since I was never able to say when my seizures would start or how long they would last. Having recently started voluntary work and working on my books and other projects my support worker struggled to arrange time with me.

An ambulance was called out to me at least twice a month. I would be either brought back home in an ambulance due to others calling them out or end up in A&E. On each call out everyone would raise concern about me being out on my own. However I could go days or a few weeks without incident and I would only ever end up in accident and emergency about twice a year either because I had taken myself in; or I because I had been admitted by ambulance due to my injuries. Otherwise I would sign the release form and get the bus back home or continue with whatever it was I was doing before the seizure occurred, unless the paramedics took me home. It wasn't until later in the twenty first century or getting into 2015 I found it difficult to avoid A&E.

I would remember what I did afterwards or recall the event a few minutes later but I could just as easily forget which could be just as annoying to me as it was to others.
I asked a neighbour if he could put a few things in his freezer whilst my fridge freezer was defrosting. However when I returned to collect those

items, I did not recognise my milk; I nearly denied that the milk was mine. Not only that, I then proceeded to put my butter in the freezer and then totally forgot about it until the following day and I then thought I had left it at my neighbours. When I went to London not only did I nearly get off the train at the wrong stop but I totally forgot where I was after I had a seizure on the train. If it was not for another passenger I would never have made it to my friend's wedding in goring by the sea.

I can recall certain events but I find my life rather sketchy. I have conversations with people and no memory of the actual event until half way through the conversation or hours later when the actual event returns. Sometimes it can take days for actual memory to return. I suffer with short term memory which means I can put things down and lose them, forget where I leave things, and forget a person's name shortly after being introduced. I also forget faces and have always forgotten the third item on a list. I have poor sense of direction and struggle to recall a conversation with someone I may have had six months down the line. Having had the intracranial EEG has only made me more aware of my memory difficulties although I find myself having to explain to people just how my memory affects me. I guess people only assume my memory difficulties are acceptable to people of a certain age. I have struggled getting a publisher for my children's book and getting some support from various charities. Working with others has its own difficulties, family and friends do not understand me, I find I am limited to friends who understand and have little patience. I also found that I have struggled to get the right people to support me with my books. I found I was invited to a wedding down south and though I felt I was treated well, there were many who had their own opinions when I shared my experience. Some felt I was used, others felt I did not treat the woman as she expected. I helped out with the venue, gave her a signed copy of my poetry book, paid for the meal and her breakfast the day before the wedding, assisted in helping out and looking after her house on the night of the wedding. I offered to send copies of the wedding photos to her and put them on canvas. However I found that when I returned home I had been deleted from her friends list and everyone I met had removed me from their friends list. When I checked my phone for the wedding photos I found all but one photo had been removed. To this day I am unsure why this happened. However I did enjoy the experience and remain eternally grateful. It was a pleasure meeting her and her family.

Over the years I have been invited to many weddings, however due to my epilepsy I have had some difficulty getting there. Often it is not just the travelling to various locations i have to take into consideration. Often it is the fear of having a attack whilst on my way or whilst at the event. If it wasn't the fact that I often come round surrounded by paramedics or in ambulances knowing that i made the effort to turn up to events. I would have no problem attending. However not every experience is like the ones I've discussed.

Chapter Seventeen

My Campaign

As my work with the insurance company only lasted for two and a half years and I found myself feeling frustrated and disillusioned being out of work, I started to focus more on the charities I was finding myself involved with. I felt that if I could educate and change the perspective of how other people who do not suffer with epilepsy view people like me; then perhaps the next time I entered a work setting my experience might be different. I wanted to eradicate stigma, change attitudes and hopefully encourage a happy medium or more tolerance in working environments. My campaigns would not just be about educating others and raising awareness, I found myself being part of other things too.

I felt frustrated that I was finding getting work and keeping a job difficult despite friends and family telling me that it was ok not to work. I have always worked since leaving school and even while I was at school I used to baby sit and do paper rounds or help my mum out or my grandmother out with cleaning jobs. I found I actually enjoyed the social aspect of a working environment and felt it was good from a mental health perspective and helped my anxiety. So I could not understand why anyone would want to put someone out of work and encourage a person not to work unless they were physically unable go out to work. Perhaps others felt that with my condition being the way it was, I was safer not working. To me anyone could work regardless of their condition. Just because my disability was on the inside until I collapsed, fainted or had a seizure didn't give people the right to assume that I was capable or incapable of meeting targets? I wanted people to see that epilepsy was not just collapsing on the floor and a person's body going into spasm with limbs jerking.

I know how to assess the dangers to myself and do not mind working with other charities and organisations to help educate them on the different illnesses and medical conditions and similarities, if this helps stamps out ignorance and helps raise awareness in order to help others. However, I am constantly coming up against ignorance and discrimination where ever I go. I sometimes feel like I am stepping back in time rather than moving forward.

When someone is treated "differently" that person's confidence can also be affected. People see the visible convulsions or tonic clonic seizures. Yet no one see's the inside of the person, their personality or what that person is capable of.

I addition to the work I used to do to help my mum, I also went to brownies and girl guides and trained in first aid with Saint John's ambulance all before I started college. I did voluntary work with Barnardo's and many other day centres whilst still at school. I was working by the age of fifteen and holding down three jobs plus a full time college course and going out with my friends three nights a week by the age of eighteen. Yet people

160

assume that because you have epilepsy you cannot work without support. You cannot go out alone; you basically have twenty four hour support. This was a pattern that was a common assumption in many parts of the UK.

I do not want to sound racist but I found I had a more positive experience living in Scotland, than in England. If it was not for financial reasons I would have stayed there. I found that in Scotland there was a much more positive attitude. I found it easier to get work and keep hold of my job. Back in the northwest of England I got the impression people wanted to wrap me up in cotton wool. Was it out of fear, lack of education or because society in England is so target driven they preferred you to be mentally and physically well before you worked in any organisation or business? I was not allowed to work on my own or front of house and people treated me as though I was a fragile child.

If a person with epilepsy is covered with cotton wool then they do not have a life. If they are told that they can't do that or not to go there or get involved in that then that is where the fear and anxiety will come from. You cannot stop a seizure from occurring just like you cannot predict a fall or road accident. So why would you treat a person with epilepsy any different from someone with depression?

The fact that people do not seem to be aware epilepsy and different type of seizures led me to become more involved with campaigns and charities. I lobbied MP's and wrote to and emailed police, local councillors and schools. I wrote to as many celebrities as possible in order to raise awareness of epilepsy and mental health. I also wanted to raise awareness about the impact epilepsy and mental health has on family and friends besides the social impact or how isolating they can be.

This is something I am still keen to keep doing and find as many alternative creative ways of campaigning and raising awareness as possible, as I feel at times people do not seem to care or if they do, there is still stigma attached. I often find that even today there are still people out there that have no idea what to do if a person has a seizure or how to react if a person was to come into the work place. With the government wanting people off income support and back into work I really do not understand why charities have had their funding cut when they are getting a surge in disabled people getting in touch for support.

It would make more sense to educate employers and have charities working together with a range of services, but this has not been the case and in all my years of experience I found my life was easier just after leaving school. I left school in 1994 and found work easy. I was able to hold down a variety of jobs whilst going to college. I never experienced stigma and discrimination again in the work place until I left Scotland.

In between working on the children's book and looking for a publisher or another alternative for my second poetry book I found myself still working on campaigns. Rather than getting involved with charities directly, I would often get more involved with charities, groups and other campaigners through the various social networking sites online. I found the internet was a useful tool for both my campaign work and my books although I often found that I opened my self-up to regular viruses and problems with my computer. Sometimes I felt that I was open to hackers or that people online were watching what was going on as the campaigns were often made public. I never knew of anyone else who had so many problems with the computer other than those I knew online who were openly campaigning and using Facebook and other social networking sights to raise awareness and run campaigns.

My cause

I work hard out of love, Sometimes though I strive,
I campaign; I feel it isn't good enough.
Love is what drives me, love is what I feel.
Though even my cause is what is so real.
I do it out of love.

Through the stalls, the charities,
The fundraising too,
My cause keeps me hooked.
Because one day, someone will see,
Someone will hear, someone will come,
Because one day my cause will come first,
My cause will be heard.
One day someone will see me,
Notice my hard work.
See my cause for what it is worth.
Notice how real and true,
Notice the importance my cause is to you.

My cause, though I work hard out of love,

Though I strive to raise awareness,

My cause never feels good enough.

Through stalls, through my campaign,

The reason for my cause, so personal to me,

Well I do it out of love, in the hope of a cure,

Well I guess the purpose of my cause keeps me hooked.

Through stalls, the charities too,

Just watch one day my cause might just come to you.

I smile, I weep, I think about my cause as I sleep.

I get frustrated as I send emails and await their return.

Through magazines and newsletters there is so much more to my cause,

So much more I can learn.

Mps I approach, conferences I attend,

With hope of some interest and one been a friend.

Support groups and meetings I try to embrace,

Magazines I bye with hast, and newspapers too,

With the hope of some news of my cause,

Perhaps there is a breakthrough for which I will applause.

If only someone would see my cause.

Another Way 2011 www.amazon.com/author/jolenemodd

I wrote this poem back in 2010 after I started becoming frustrated with all the charity work I was becoming involved in. I had done extensive research on various websites, asking doctors, consultants and a variety of others questions about my condition and various other forms of epilepsy including looking into the variety of support and help available. I was doing research into epilepsy and alternative treatments on websites that were been screened from other countries that I found to be ahead of the UK. I started getting more creative with my poems. I thought that perhaps I could combine the charity work with my other ambition which was to publish my poetry. May be I could use my poems to raise awareness of epilepsy and get others to listen? Though I had experienced a number of problems with my computer I succeeded in getting my first poetry book published in March 2010 through a self-publishing company although I was not happy with the result. The problems with my computer meant that I relied on the publishing company to edit and proof read my book for me and convert my disk to the latest software.

Unfortunately that did not happen and my first book turned into a disaster which was not the result I was looking for. However it was my first experience and my first ever poetry book to be published. I found I took better care of my computer after that experience. I started publishing my poetry online sharing my work with others every epilepsy awareness month and writing poetry that was related to the various campaigns.

I had been to Westminster back in 2009 and this also turned out to be a particular bad year for me. It was the year I got back on route with the decision to look into the option of neuro surgery, the year so many famous people and icons passed away either as a result of drugs, alcohol or brain related or neurological conditions such as epilepsy.

It started with David Cameron's son who passed away I am not sure if epilepsy claimed Ivan Cameron in the end or if it was simply his "time" as Ivan had other disabilities as well. Awareness was raised but not many people were taking notice, cancer was on the increase and seemed to be claiming a lot of celebrities' lives. More celebrities came forward about their epilepsy but nothing more was said or done until Jet Travolta, John Travolta's son passed away in the bath after a seizure. I thought may be the government and council would have looked into the importance of installing free showers in council properties where they were needed however I was still turned down on two separate occasions as my flat I was told was unsuitable due to its size and structure for a wet room.

I realised I would have to pay for one myself and the plumbing too, I can imagine the row should anything have happened to me while I was still occupying the flat. Regardless of my concerns or anyone else's I knew I was not alone in my quest for a shower or wet room, I knew there were others just like me with similar problems and issues all over the UK. Getting back to my campaign I felt like I was still often talking to the brick wall.

I would make the use of the internet often, getting involved with twitter, face book, various charities and their websites. I became a chair person for our local support group and would often attend meetings and conferences at the local hospital, get involved with campaigns, approach MPs, councillors, local police officers on the streets, security staff while they were working, schools, community centres, chat to the local fire services, get involved with various other charities, approach members of the public, put up posters, you name it I was doing it.

Everything I did was with the intention of raising awareness and letting people know there was no need to fear their condition. I wanted people to ask me questions, I wanted to educate people about epilepsy and erase the stigmas and fears that surround us.

However nothing I ever did ever seemed to be good enough, every month I would attend the local meetings and groups expecting to see more people turn up only to be greeted by the same faces. Subs were stopped as there was no point in taking money as we weren't spending anything, and we didn't see the point in trying to entice people into the groups by saying there would be a speaker coming this month as no one seemed to be talking an interest in my wall or twitter feed anyway.

If I couldn't get people to attend my group by offering free tea and coffee or free biscuits what was going to get them past their front doors? I even went round people's houses collecting people at one point, and I would phone people up a week before reminding them about the group or knock on their doors or text them two days before and ask them were they coming.

I even got to that stage where I was offering to sort out peoples bus passes, benefits and housing issues. A specialist nurse once informed me that I was doing the job of a social worker yet I was the one who needed a social worker for my own issues. Twice I had a go at running my own business but was never successful either because of my epilepsy or because I didn't have the life experience or a business partner willing to support me. Well if life experience is what people are after maybe they should think about my life experience after reading my book?

To me disability is a state of mind there are many ways around it, anyone can work or hold down a job, I lost mine because of attitude, stigmas, fears and perceptions and may be a lack in understanding. My aim by writing this book is to change that and show you that there is nothing to fear and there is always something out there for you regardless of who you are. Never give up. I have not, I am just taking some time out to regroup and sort my health out and I have every intention of going back to work. Working with others is something I enjoy doing, I always wanted to run a workshop and a group and I don't see how having epilepsy should get in the way of that. Maybe I have just been going down one or two wrong paths; or the paths I have taken are the paths I needed to take to get to where I am today. Writing my books and publishing them is another way of fulfilling another dream or ambition of mine.

I wanted to raise awareness and the way I watched others do it didn't seem to be making an impact, I wanted to do it in a way that people would listen where attitudes could change and where people would realise that they could be more positive, those living with any disability; not just epilepsy but anyone regardless of their disability would know they could go out there and achieve anything and deal with it. May be putting up posters, writing to the BBC, the MPs and the Primary Care Trust (PCT)was not the direction to go in, maybe there was a better way of getting my message across? Though this method appealed to me at the time.

It horrified me to learn that like many other people living with epilepsy I was been compared to someone with a learning disability, mental health or illness and perhaps that was why I was not getting as far in my career as I was expecting . One in three people with a learning disability have epilepsy probably because brain disorder and people being born prematurely are more likely to develop other medical conditions - epilepsy being just one of them. At the same time epilepsy is just as common as migraine and so is mental health. A high proportion of people with learning disabilities and epilepsy find it difficult to control their epilepsy and they probably also have migraines and depression which is a mental illness. Does that mean we should treat them any differently to the rest of the population?

1 in 131 of people have epilepsy which means that epilepsy is a common condition. Therefore more money and emphasis should be going into research not stigmatising people and treating them differently. The brain is a sensitive organ and causes of epilepsy involve head injury, birth trauma, stroke, brain tumour, infections such as meningitis, encephalitis, alcohol and drugs and epilepsy can even be inherited. In 65% of cases of epilepsy the cause is unknown. Epilepsy is the second most common neurological condition in the UK after migraine and people do not get treated any different because they suffer migraine attacks.

So far I feel like my journey has been a rollercoaster. I'm still no further towards achieving my goals, understanding myself or even raising awareness for people with epilepsy. Although the BBC and other channels often issue a warning when there are flashing lights or flash photography before the screen starts flashing thanks to a campaign I was part of. The police now are more aware of epilepsy and what to do if a person is unconscious or unresponsive and there is more awareness of epilepsy and the causes due to various campaigns that various charities and organisations have run and the work we do as part of a team. It is still difficult to get paid work if you have a neurological condition although voluntary work is becoming easier. There are more people however now working for them.

As well as sorting out my health I have been busy with the charity work and so far, other than a poem I have included I have not really mentioned the work I have done for charity.

I'm not entirely sure how long I have been a member of Epilepsy Action although I know I was a member when I moved up to Scotland in 2001. I was aware of them and the forum on their website. The epilepsy forum has been very supportive, especially since I decided to go down the surgery route with the hospital in London. Mostly, the only contact I have had on the forum is through the discussion board or by email.

I have met many people with epilepsy and other neurological conditions through website forums or social networks such as Facebook or through hospitals or support groups. Through meeting these people I have found strength, courage and inspiration.

These friendships have helped me to cope with my own epilepsy and find new ways to get involved with charities. One difficulty I found was getting voluntary work, despite coming out of work myself and passing three CRB checks I was unable to get a part time voluntary post because of my epilepsy. So I took it up on myself to get involved with various other charities and campaigns to help raise awareness and support others with various disabilities including epilepsy.

In doing this I found I gained a lot of support and information that I too needed. Though I learned that despite encouraging a lot of famous people to come forward there was still a lot of ignorance and stigma surrounding epilepsy. I found people seemed to get further ahead in their careers if they did better in their English and maths and remained quiet about their medical condition. Once someone was claiming benefits from the state it was difficult to get off government hand-outs and into work, and if a person's seizures were difficult to control then they risked being treated (by most people) like a child or as someone who was stupid or incapable. It was very difficult to get away from this stigma once the stigma was attached. I found campaign work and research helped though it often felt as though I was going round in circles; and every achievement or accomplishment I made was a slow process. This was the frustrating part that I often experienced which did affect my mood and often resulted in the feelings of anxiety. I found therapy, training and group support often helped me through this process although it was challenging to stay positive and go with the flow even believing that there was a reason for everything and that I would get there in the end. It was not easy.

I am still very angry that despite all the hard work I put in and all the research I have done into epilepsy; I have not succeeded in changing much. I feel that the UK is still behind some countries. It amazes me how we are still in a lot of debt yet we are living in a society where people are more materialistic and interested in money than in working together as a community and helping others. As a spiritual person I wonder what it will take in order to make a person see or view the world or a situation differently.

Sometimes my memories are much more vivid and visual and only recalled with the help of music, sometimes with the help of pictures or by listening to other people's experiences. I have found since my surgery in 2011 it is my memories of childhood that are the strongest. In 2014 I was invited to a friend's wedding which was basically a Facebook romance which blossomed with the help of Epilepsy Action. I set up my Facebook page when my own support group originally closed down in 2009 and I wanted to stay connected with others who had similar problems. I found myself connecting with people all over the world. Not only was I connecting with other individuals with neurological conditions, I was connecting with people with mental health conditions, other support groups and individuals who had family members and friends with various other conditions. I was not just using my Facebook group to raise awareness and run campaigns but to educate and support people too.

In November 2013 I was invited to an epilepsy meet up in London. I had the opportunity to sell some of my books to raise money for Epilepsy Action and to meet up with likeminded people.

I found voluntary work has also been a good experience for me, working in groups was a good way of raising awareness and working with people with various other disabilities. However not only was it a learning curve for me but an experience. I found not only was this a good experience for my memory skills but my own creativity.

Chapter Eighteen

Self-Employment

As mentioned in My Story, over the years I have made many attempts to set up my own business.

When I lived in Glasgow I was involved in a small business gateway course to enable me to set up groups and run various groups and support groups. I was already involved in studying the first year of an advanced diploma course in therapeutic counselling, had gained experience working with vulnerable young adults, drug and alcohol and homeless people. I felt I wanted to do more with my qualification. Having had a go of running groups and workshops for small businesses and other organisations I knew this was something I wanted to do. When I moved back to Manchester I knew that for insurance purposes and due to my epilepsy it would be better for myself if I had a business partner. Though the business I set up in Glasgow was unsuccessful due to my epilepsy it gave me experience and the confidence and determination to continue once I had my health sorted.

When I left the insurance company I went on a second course to try again at setting up my business, this time with a business partner. We were looking at setting up a holistic therapy centre. We had gone as far as researching the venue, pricing the venue, looking into contracts and advertising costs. However my business partner dropped out before we signed the contract which meant I had to revise my business venture. Due to health and safety I needed someone more experienced than me in order to set up the centre. Once the business was set up I could then apply for insurance and finish of the relevant courses that were needed in order to make the business a success. But when my business partner dropped out without word or warning and went off to work for an established business, we never spoke again afterwards. I found I was hit by the recession and the bank loan I took out I ended up investing in my books and using the money to survive on while I worked on plan b. I went into business on my own as no one could take my books away. I found myself self-publishing my first poetry book and looking into ways in which I could overcome my dyslexia, memory problems and epilepsy without the negativity from those who looked at my condition as too much of a concern for someone wanting to go self-employed. I wrote to many different self-publishing companies and in the end selected one, however I was never really happy with my choice. I found I learned a great deal about the publishing industry. It gave me more encouragement and determination to look at other ways I could do things. With my second book, I was able to network with others, use the links and friends I had made in the past and use the internet in order to find other ways of reducing the cost. I sold more books by doing more research and networking than I had done previously when I published my first book. As much as I was impatient and found having lots of books in my spare room quite depressing I found that over time I learned new ways to get my name known. The more well-known I was the more books I sold. I was too afraid to spend money in the first two years on advertising as I was unsure of the risk and how going it alone would affect me. I had approached many publishers over the years and the many knock backs started to impact on my confidence. So when my editor suggested trying again I was a little sceptical. At the same time looking into print on demand cost money and self-publishing companies were even more expensive. I had already had one bad experience due to a lack of communication with my first book and

I did not want to repeat it. I did not want to start making phone calls and give in to pressure selling and so I was considering going it alone with my other books and hoping someone would notice me. Although I was growing impatient and I noticed how the pressure I was putting on myself was starting to affect my depression.

Focusing on my children's book was no better. After I had found an illustrator and graphic designer I thought my book was now ready. I now needed to approach an actor and felt that working with someone I knew well would be a lot easier than going through the phone book. I found a friend who was now a struggling actor living back with his sister who was an artist. It was quite exciting having him come to meet me to work on my children's book. I met my friend at the rail station and even bought a sofa bed for him to sleep on. The following day I took him down to the studio where we worked on the children's book. Afterwards all that was needed was for the illustrator and graphic designer to finish the book, or so I thought. It turned out that the children's book proved to be as challenging as the poetry books I was working on but at least the poetry books were in print and packed in boxes in my spare bedroom. What I thought was a straight forward journey; a passion and dream I enjoyed since childhood, turned into a stressful few years. I had already given up on my first children's book, which was a children's adventure about a flamingo with anxiety and how the bird coped. I had a pile of books from a publishing company which were unsellable and a second pile of books which were a massive improvement on the first but were just sitting there. Now I had a children's book with which the costs were mounting but I was starting to wonder if the loan I had taken out was worth it. Soon the bank were asking me if I wanted to increase my loan. I found that I had to refuse as I was not making any money in the first place.

I started to wonder if self-publishing and writing my own books were a good investment; book stores and music stores all around me were closing down and the only place where I could sell was the internet. The only way for a book to be found was if someone searched for it. In order for someone to search for the book people needed to know it was there and advertising costs online were quite high. I had already paid £95 to my fan story website for three months' advertising but it made no difference. I regularly used Facebook and Twitter account although my friends and family wanted my books for free. I had already made a start on donating books to libraries and signed up to ALCS, The Society of Authors and the Poetry Society but there was little feedback. It was not until May 2013; two years after I had self-published "Another way", signed up to the British library public lending rights and spent a year donating to various libraries across the uk that my hard work finally paid off. I had taken out a five thousand pound loan to invest in my books and having invested a huge part of my savings and loan in my passion I had started to become disillusioned. But then ALCS accepted and registered both my poetry books, both my poetry books were now registered with the British library and I now started to wonder if my hard feelings towards the self-publishing company were incorrect. I had spent over two thousand pounds on my first poetry book over three years. In that time I had only sold twelve books. Although I knew my ambition would take time I felt that in three years I should have made more progress. However, when my business advisor started to become concerned, I began to struggle with my children's book. I started to wonder if my career would ever take off. I often watched other authors promoting their books and talking to presenters discussing best sellers on TV shows. I wondered why none of my books were on those shows. I knew I was at a disadvantage with my dyslexia and epilepsy. However I had been campaigning since the age of fifteen so what was I doing wrong? Perhaps I should have stuck to writing for a hobby and not allowed the job centre to have led me on? When I came out of work I made my own assumption that I could actually do something for myself. I knew self-employment was never going to be the main source of income but I succeeded in fulfilling my dream of writing my books. I did eventually return to work and overcame my fears of working. I did of course have further surgery to come although I actually did enjoy writing.

I guess it was never going to be easy I was not going to find a job for life and my writing career was never going to be an easy one. Every week I would try to add a new chapter to this autobiography though I often found it turning into another diary. In addition I was in the process of writing my children's book and my second poetry book when my computer was hit by a number of viruses which meant starting all over again. Luckily I had backed up my work on disk though the disk was not compatible with the new software. I could still at least go back to my original work when starting over. I would eventually use a range of means to back up my work though it was often frustrating and time consuming. I would go on to have a number of problems with my PC and would find that as my memory declined I would struggle with the latest technology. I preferred floppy disk though it never really stored that much memory. I did eventually get used to memory stick though I often found I got frustrated with the computers and many forms of laptops and mobiles. I still craved for the older versions of technology that I could cope with.

Eventually I got used to different forms of technology although it still proved frustrating when dealing with publishers, illustrators and in the world of writing generally. I could never keep up with the different methods and levels of communication and technology that everyone was using. I struggled with different styles of learning and often found not everyone understood my memory issues. I still found ignorance and lack of communication in the land of publication. I did eventually succeed in writing my children's book and ended up buying a laptop which contained all the information I needed. I found that as information came through from the publishers my computer was automatically upgraded. However in order to keep up I spent more time upgrading my computer and working on my laptop than I did doing much else! The children's book became a journey of its own and while at the time it was a stressful experience it created the desired effect that I wanted.

I always knew that I had a problem with my literacy skills so finding a publisher who would look at my work without expecting me to have an English degree would be difficult. I decided to look into self-publishing once more.

As mentioned before, I had contacted many publishers, however when I returned to the UK I found my letters had all been sent back to me; some recommending self-publishing companies and others with hints and tips on how to present a manuscript. I was starting to feel depleted and self-publishing looked like the only way forward. However, it was an expensive option. I could not cope with anymore rejections so decided to put my books to one side for now. Perhaps someday I would publish a book and set up a business but for now I had my epilepsy to get under control especially now I was back out of work. However as a hobby I continued to write poetry.

In 2013 I found I was progressing with my poetry books and my children's book. I had an opportunity to republish my first poetry book with another self-publishing company in London or I could republish the book myself using the printing service I used for my second poetry book. I also was making progress with my children's book. An illustrator I had found on Twitter had now finished illustrating my children's book. I felt I was making progress with my writing career since I now had some of my poetry books in two local shops and was about to do my first book signing.

I was now involved in two organisations and was able to raise awareness of epilepsy using the internet and had an opportunity to get involved with local organisations. I felt I was making some progress.

I am continuing with my writing career, in the hope that more of my work becomes published and I can use my work to raise awareness of my cause.

Conclusion

There really is no clear conclusion, as my story and my journey is still ongoing. However my research and experiences of Epilepsy have helped me to form some conclusions as to what needs to be done in the future.

- Epilepsy is usually diagnosed in children and people over 65 years of age, although it can affect anyone at any time.

- There are **50 million** people living with epilepsy worldwide.

- In the UK around **30%** of people living with epilepsy are in what is called drug resistant epilepsy. Whereby for the sufferers medication does not work or is inadequate. Treatment such as the vagus nerve stimulation or neuro surgery helps but is not always a cure.

- The underlying **cause** of epilepsy is also a mystery along with a cure which so far is still being researched.

- Scientific research is also expensive along with medication which comes with many different side effects.

- Depression, anxiety and weight loss or weight gain cannot always be linked to epilepsy but like epilepsy have many underlying causes and cannot be treated with drugs or diet alone. I have tried them all even looked into various therapies, such as Reiki, acupuncture, massage, stress and anxiety management, counselling and various diets.

Perceptions and Stigma

Society's understanding of Epilepsy is poor though there are many books and papers published. This is due to lack of information, education and awareness which in turn creates fear and ultimately stigma. Though 2016 has seen a lot of information out in the media which I hope will lead to change.

According to NHS England Prevention is better than cure.

This can result in barriers to employment, social exclusion and unnecessary calls to the emergency services. This could be improved through, and TV programmes, further training and awareness is leading to a shift in culture.

- Introducing education about hidden disabilities at an early age through primary schools.
- Educating employers about how to deal with an epileptic employee, and ensuring protective measures are in place such as flexible working and stress free environments.
- Increasing awareness of epilepsy through the media and community information processes.
- Encouraging people to talk about it.

Medical Research and Treatment

There is already a great deal of research being carried out, but more needs to be done, in particular with regard to triggers and causes of epilepsy. Improvements could be made in the following areas:-

- Communication between medical personnel, patients and carers.
- Looking at holistic ways of managing the condition such as diet.
- Whether alternative therapies can be of benefit.

- Looking at other methods rather than automatically putting someone on medication which can have side-effects.

In 2013 the European Commission recognized the need for better care for people with neurological disorders; they still had some way to go in order to stamp out stigma and discrimination. More awareness was needed but it was a sign that all that campaign work was showing progress. MNDs include a number of disorders, including epilepsy, schizophrenia, Alzheimer's disease and depression, and affect about 700 million people each year, according to the World Health Organization.

Since 2007, the European Commission has dedicated less than 2 billion Euros to brain research through a framework of funding bodies known as FP7. It now plans to replace FP7 with a new framework called Horizon, which will run from 2014-2020 and will have a much larger budget for neurological research. Progress in research will not be achieved by countries in isolation, but through carefully considered international plans, for which each country will have different priorities. Some of the research areas that neurologists have already highlighted are: brain structure and function, ontogenetic, disease prevention and early diagnosis. The Neurological Alliance is concerned that some patients' care is adversely affected by a lack of specialist knowledge and 'haphazard' services in their local area.

Glossary

GLOSSARY

Absence Seizure –	**Petit Mal / blank spells**
Alzheimer's –	**Dementia**
Amnesia –	**forgetfulness (an inability to remember)**
Anxiety – apprehension	**A general term used to describe nervousness, fear, or**
Auras-	**A warning that occurs before a seizure**
Atonic Seizure –	**person slumps to the ground but recovers quickly**
Atrosphy –	**wasting or loss of muscle tissue due to damage**
Autism – early childhood development.	**A mental or neurological condition, present from that affects a person's**
Allergic reactions	**Can be a possible side effect of medications**
Attitudes	**Historical set of beliefs ,Stigmas, fear of the unknown,** a settled way of thinking or feeling , an opinion about something or someone.
Anesthetic patient	**Local Anesthetic is something surgeons use to sedate a** during a operation.
Brand	**Type of product manufactured by a company**
Cryptogenic "hidden") Epilepsy –	**from the Greek word "kryptos," meaning** **is epilepsy with no obvious cause.**

Depression – can cause anxiety,	The possibility of a seizure at any time or place embarrassment, or anger. These and other negative emotions may bring on depression. Hormone levels can also play a role in triggering depression in people with epilepsy. Researchers found that low estrogen levels are common those with depression.
Drop-down Seizure –	**Atonic Seizures**
Dyslexia –	**known as reading disorder, trouble with reading** **despite normal intelligence**
EEG –	**An electroencephalogram, a recording of brain**
Generic	Relating to a class or group of things
Hippocampus –	**The part of the brain** the brain, thought to be the centre of emotion, memory, and the autonomic nervous system.
Homonymous	is the loss of half of the field of view on the same s idle in both eyes
Hemianopia –	visual field loss
Idiopathic Simple Partial	**Not all seizures occurring during adult life are due to epilepsy** **Epilepsy – Many are acute symptomatic** **seizure which must be recognized to avoid inappropriate antiepileptic drugs been used. (idiopathic)**
Motor Cortex –	**One of the brain areas most involved in controlling these voluntary movements**
Myoclonic Seizure –	**brief shock-like jerks**
NEAD –	**Non epileptic Attack disorder**

184

Neuro-surgery –   surgery performed on the nervous system,
                        especially the brain and spinal cord

Neutropenia –   **A condition that effects the white blood cells**

Neutrophils –   **white blood count**

OCD –   **Obsessive compulsive disorder**

Occipital Lobe –   **The back of the brain**

Partial Seizure –   **Partial   seizures   are   split   into   two   main**
categories;

                     simple   partial   seizures   and   complex   partial
seizures

                     in partial seizures a small part of the lobes may
be affected

Photo-Sensitive
Epilepsy –   **a person is effected by flashing lights, strobe**
lighting

                     which can bring on a migraine or seizure.

Syncope –   **Temporary loss of consciousness caused by a fall**
in blood pressure,

                     fainting attack or temporary loss of
                     consciousness with a fast recovery

Temporal Lobe –   **Part of the brain**

Tonic Clonic Seizure – **This type is what most people think of when they**
                     hear the word "seizure." An   older term for
                     them is "grand mal.

Vagus Nervous   **cranial nerves, An Which supplies the heart,**
                     lungs, upper digestive tract,   and   other   organs
                     of the chest and abdomen.

Further reading

Further reading : N Engl J Med 1998;338:20-24. CHADWICK D. (2000) Seizures and epilepsy after traumatic brain injury. Oxford Medical Dictionary ,
Lancet 2000;355:334-336. FOY PM, COPELAND GP, SHAW MDM. Incidence of post-operative seizures. Acta Neurochir 1981;55:13-24. London ULCH, Glyn Volans and heather Wiseman Bsc. Barry J Gibb. The British Medical Association , www.epilepsyaction.co.uk. ANNEGERS JF, HAUSER WA, COAN SP, ROCCA WA.

DISCLAIMER

It should be noted that the medications mentioned in this book and the descriptions of their side effects are personal to the Author.

Any comments made about their use and consequences is in no way meant to be detrimental to the manufacturers. For others suffering with   epilepsy the drugs mentioned may have been used successfully to control the condition.

Useful links and organisations

www.epilepsyaction.co.uk   www.scottishambulance.com

https://www.**bhf**.org.**uk**   020 7554 0376 heart start

https://www.**bma**.org.**uk**

www.**epilepsy**.com

www.young**epilepsy**.org.uk

www.**epilepsy**scotland.org.uk

www.educationscotland.gov.uk/resources

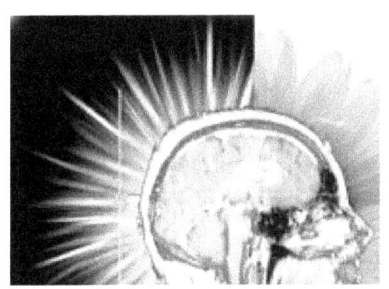

(C) Copy Right J Modd 2016

www.ingramcontent.com/pod-product-compliance
Lightning Source LLC
Chambersburg PA
CBHW051503170526
45166CB00001B/365